T0256254

Occupational Therapy
with
Borderline Patients

Occupational Therapy with Borderline Patients

Diane Gibson, MS, OTR
Editor

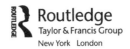

Routledge
Taylor & Francis Group
New York   London

Occupational Therapy with Borderline Patients has also been published as *Occupational Therapy in Mental Health,* Volume 3, Number 3, Fall 1983.

First pubished by

The Haworth Press, Inc., 28 East 22 Street, New York, NY 10010

This edition published 2012 by Routledge

Routledge
Taylor & Francis Group
711 Third Avenue
New York, NY 10017

Routledge
Taylor & Francis Group
2 Park Square, Milton Park
Abingdon, Oxon OX14 4RN

Library of Congress Cataloging in Publication Data
Main entry under title:

Occupational therapy with borderline patients.

"Has also been published as Occupational therapy in mental health, volume 3, number 3, fall 1983"—T. p. verso.
Includes bibliographical references.
1. Personality, Disorders of—Treatment—Addresses, essays, lectures.
2. Occupational therapy—Addresses, essays, lectures. 3. Mentally ill—Rehabilitation—Addresses, essays, lectures. I. Gibson, Diane.
[DNLM: 1. Personality disorders—Rehabilitation. 2. Occupational therapy. W1 0C601N v.3 no.3 / WM 190 015]
RC554.O25   1983   616.89   83-13008
ISBN 0-86656-262-1

Occupational Therapy with Borderline Patients

Occupational Therapy in Mental Health
Volume 3, Number 3

CONTENTS

SUSAN CLEARY SCHWARTZ, OTR, *Program Coordinator, Inpatient Psychiatry Unit, Pacific Medical Center, San Francisco, California*

DIANE SHAPIRO, MA, OTR, *Director of Therapeutic Activities, The New York Hospital—Cornell Medical Center Westchester Division, White Plains, New York*

JANE SLAYMAKER, MA, OTR, FAOTA, *Associate Professor, Department of Occupational Therapy, University of Florida, Gainesville, Florida*

FRANKLIN STEIN, PhD, OTR, *Director, Occupational Therapy Program, University of Wisconsin, Milwaukee*

MARY SAVAGE STOWELL, MS, OTR, *Coordinator, Day Treatment Program, Grossmont Hospital, LaMesa, California*

ELIZABETH TIFFANY, MEd, OTR, FAOTA, *Associate Professor, Department of Occupational Therapy, Temple University, Philadelphia, Pennsylvania*

JOYCE WARD, MS, OTR, *Chair, Occupational Therapy Department, San Jose State University, San Jose, California*

SUSAN WILLIAMS, MA, OTR, *Project Director, ISIS, San Francisco, California*

ELIZABETH YERXA, EdD, OTR, FAOTA, *Chairperson, Occupational Therapy Program, University of Southern California, Downey, California*

Foreword

Borderline patients are widely recognized as extremely difficult to treat given their self-destructive and maladaptive interpersonal relations, which, when coupled with their typical defenses of splitting, projective identification and omnipotence, can leave clinicians feeling vulnerable and impotent.

Considerable literature is now available regarding the developmental origins and personality structure of borderline patients, and an understanding of their dynamics appears absolutely necessary for effective treatment. However, scant information is available to assist mental health professionals in managing these patients' severe behavioral and emotional maladjustment, their extraordinary vacillation between clinging dependency and hostile attacks and their overwhelming sense of aloneness and rejection. Furthermore, almost no articles have been published which offer guidelines to treat the borderline patient in occupational therapy or in the other activity therapies.

The manuscripts in this publication have been chosen to offer the front line clinician an opportunity to review current knowledge in the theoretical concepts, the management, and the design of activity groups for borderline patients.

Dr. Charles Peters, in *An Historical Review of the Borderline Concept,* traces initial early attempts to understand this puzzling disorder. Many formulations, such as preschizophrenia, ambulatory schizophrenia, pseudoneurotic schizophrenia, and "as-if" personality suggest the confusion and concern regarding this condition. The object relations theorists are noted as the most recent and perhaps the most valuable theorists in that they stress understanding of personality structure rather than symptomatology. They postulate that the genesis of the borderline phenomenon rests in the lack of separation-individuation of the child from the mother in the rapprochement or "terrible twos" stage of infant development. Fixation at this stage prevents the integration of good and bad representations within the perception of self and within the perception of significant others. The inability to affectively separate self from nonself and to integrate good and bad representations provide the basis for splitting, the borderline patient's common defense which profoundly affects all aspects of his/her functioning.

Two articles, written by occupational therapists, address the translation of theory into prescriptions for purposeful activity. Both are valuable and useful to practicing occupational therapists since they offer critical new thinking in determining guidelines for the care of the borderline patient.

Gail Goodman's article, *Occupational Therapy Treatment: Interventions with Borderline Patients,* notes the difficulties these patients experience in selecting and carrying out work and leisure pursuits. Although the borderline patient does not suffer diminution in intellectual abilities, his/her struggle to maintain an independent self-concept sets up ongoing problems in dependent-independent issues, inability to accept criticism and an inability to sublimate drives which might lead to experiencing pleasure in activity. Goodman suggests creative-expressive media, leisure experiences, and work groups for patients dealing with anxiety producing, ambiguous, unconscious conflicts. She believes the primary therapeutic functions of the occupational therapist are to assist the borderline patient in making a choice (of activity) and to recognize when unconscious feelings are provoked. Other functions include confronting the patient's defenses and redirecting him/her to task when he/she experiences failure and resultant depression.

Cheryl Salz, in *A Theoretical Approach to the Treatment of Work Difficulties in Borderline Personalities,* traces several psychodynamic theories and emphasizes the usefulness of Kielhofner's and Burke's human occupations model. Regarding the genesis of borderline dysfunction, it is postulated that exploratory play is important to the child's emerging independence and to his ability to experience pleasure in volitionally selected activity. As the mother (in an attempt to keep the child close), thwarts exploratory play, she prevents the child's gradual assumption of developmental subsystems which normally move from exploration (pre-school) to skill competency (grade school) to role achievement (adolescence). A vicious circle is created, and the borderline individual eventually experiences inadequate habit and skill patterns, little pleasure, extreme ambivalent impulsivity and a sense of emptiness.

Through a series of interesting case studies, Salz illustrates this model in conceptualizing occupational therapy services for the borderline patient. Emphasis is placed on clear expectations in a "doing environment, one which encourages exploration of alternatives, choices and problems and one which allows safety and acceptance of failure.

Carol Kaplan, a psychiatric nurse, offers understanding and helpful intervention techniques in *Inpatient Management of the Borderline Patient,* whose acting out, destructive and manipulative behavior can "tear asunder" highly skilled clinical teams. She acknowledges that covert problems within the treatment team may be mobilized by the borderline patient and proposes means to examine team dynamics in association with typical borderline defenses. Her ideas are not only practical and helpful on an operational basis, but they also tie theory to practice in a manner which practitioners can understand.

Two articles are reprinted due to their excellence in formulating treatment of the hospitalized borderline patient. Dr. Jerry Lewis, in *Early Treatment Planning for Hospitalized Severe Borderline Patients,* outlines the stages of treatment and presents some very important thoughts about the quality and timing of confrontation. Paula Kernberg's article, *Update of Borderline Disorders in Children,* reviews this disorder as seen in children, stressing the need to recognize coexisting organicity and the value of psychoanalytically oriented therapy.

Diane Gibson, MS, OTR
Editor

An Historical Review
of the Borderline Concept

Charles P. Peters, MD

ABSTRACT. An overview of the origin and evolution of the borderline concept is presented. Relevant historical trends are identified and a framework is established on which to base further study. The works of Kraepelin, Freud, and Bleuler are seen to lay the foundation for later systems of diagnosis and classification. Early metapsychologists provided insight into the psychological dynamics of the borderline patient, while the early descriptive psychopathologists contributed significantly to our phenomenological description of this patient population. Robert Knight in the early 1950s and John Gunderson in the mid-1970s synthesized the work that preceded them. Of the recent psychostructural writings, Otto Kernberg was considered representative. Roy Grinker's research epitomized a more descriptive and empirical approach to the problem of diagnostic criteria. Family and genetic studies as well as an evolving body of pharmacological literature are briefly reviewed. DSM III and the work of Robert Spitzer are considered current endpoints in an attempt to integrate and delineate varying conceptualizations of the borderline patient.

Few areas of psychopathology have attracted as much attention in recent years as the borderline concept. Having an ambiguous origin and an often elusive evolution, the term "borderline" continues to stir feelings of bewilderment and avoidance in many clinicians. Moore and Fine (1967) gave the following definition of the word "borderline" in their glossary: "A descriptive term referring to a group of conditions which manifest both neurotic and psychotic

Dr. Peters is Assistant Director of Residency Training at the Sheppard and Enoch Pratt Hospital in Towson, Maryland and Clinical Instructor of Psychiatry at the University of Maryland, School of Medicine.

1

phenomena without fitting unequivocally into either diagnostic category.'' This article introduces the reader to the borderline concept from an historical perspective and develops a theoretical and descriptive foundation on which to build a comprehensive understanding of this pathological construct (see Figure 1).

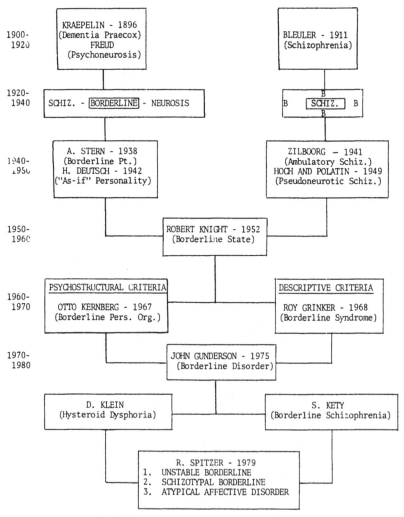

FIGURE 1. Evolution of the Borderline Concept

EARLY SYSTEMS OF DIAGNOSIS AND CLASSIFICATION

Prior to 1900, few formal systems of psychiatric classification had been developed. Attention to the major psychoses was primarily in the form of case studies.

Morel first introduced the term "dementia praecox" in 1856 when describing an adolescent patient who was originally bright and active but who gradually became withdrawn, angry, and delusional. Descriptions of "catatonia" by Kahlbaum and "hebephrenia" by Hecker followed in 1868 and 1870. It was not until the latter part of the 19th century, however, that Kraepelin attempted to synthesize these varied clinical descriptions into an orderly system of classification (Lehmann, 1975).

At the turn of the century, the term "borderline" was being used to refer to a group of individuals considered to be enemies of society and having psychopathic personalities. These were the antisocial and criminal individuals whose pathology was thought secondary to a degenerative hereditary process (Capponi, 1979). This early usage of the term lends less to our understanding of what was to follow than does an analysis of the work of Kraepelin, Freud, and Bleuler in their efforts to delineate the psychoses from the neuroses.

In his 1896 edition of the *Compendium of Psychiatry,* Kraepelin considered dementia praecox to be the major diagnostic category under which the psychotic disorders described earlier would fall. He included catatonia, hebephrenia, and paranoia as examples of dementia praecox, believing that each of these disorders had an early age of onset and a deteriorating course. Dementia praecox was distinguished from manic depressive psychosis in his 1898 paper, "The Diagnosis and Prognosis of Dementia Praecox." The major distinguishing features were again related to age of onset and course of illness. Unlike dementia praecox, Kraepelin believed that manic depressive illness began later in life and had a remitting or cyclical clinical course.

Kraepelin's definition of dementia praecox was a narrow one that made it readily distinguishable from manic depressive illness and from the psychoneurotic disorders being described concurrently by Freud.

Theoretically at least, the turn of the century saw the evolution of what seemed to be a clear nosological dichotomy of psychotic disorders on the one hand and neurotic disorders on the other. This dichotomy had hardly emerged, however, when it became clear that the matter of classification was not so simple.

Freud (1961) appreciated the problem of those patients who seemed to fall somewhere between the neuroses and the "dementia praecox" of Kraepelin. He wrote in 1913 "Often enough, when one sees a case of neurosis with hysterical or obsessional symptoms, mild in character and of short duration, a doubt which must not be overlooked arises as to whether the case may not be one of insipient dementia praecox and may not sooner or later develop well-marked signs of this disease."

Eugen Bleuler (1950) imagined the situation of the psychoses to be somewhat different from that proposed by Kraepelin. Feeling strongly that dementia praecox was far too narrow a concept, he proceeded to broaden the definition of this disorder. Bleuler considered early age of onset and deteriorating course to be unnecessarily rigid prerequisites for the diagnosis and focused instead on much less concrete criteria. Bleuler contended that a disturbance of associative thought processes, a breaking down of associative threads, was the common denominator among the major psychotic disorders. He abandoned the term dementia praecox in 1911 and renamed these patients "schizophrenic." The result of Bleuler's attempt to diagnose by inference (assuming a disruption of associative thought processes from outwardly evident signs and symptoms) was that many more patients were considered schizophrenic than had previously been the case. Indeed, patients who once seemed undiagnosable in the dementia praecox-neurosis dichotomy were now considered to be on the border of schizophrenia.

The importance of appreciating the narrow descriptive definition of schizophrenia advanced by Kraepelin and the broader, more inferential notion of this disorder described by Bleuler is that each strongly influenced the ensuing attempts to understand the "in between" patient. Those clinicians and researchers who were influenced by Kraepelin's narrow definition of schizophrenia tended to see the borderline disorder as a distinct clinical entity. Others, subscribing more willingly to the broader notion of schizophrenia as set forth by Bleuler, assumed these patients to be schizophrenic subtypes.

Two relatively distinct trends emerged in the first half of the 20th century. One trend represented the work of the metapsychologists, primarily psychoanalysts, who believed that an understanding of intrapsychic processes would shed light on the etiology and nature of the borderline disorder. The descriptive psychopathologists, in turn, focused their efforts more heavily on the behavioral and phenomenologic delineation of this patient population. Adolph Stern and Helene Deutsch were among those in the former group while Zilboorg, Hoch, and Polatin were among the latter.

THE PSYCHOANALYTIC LITERATURE: EARLY CONTRIBUTIONS

The contributions to the borderline literature by psychoanalytic writers were characterized by three relatively consistent findings. First, the patient population being described was a fairly functional one not requiring hospital treatment at the time of initial presentation. Second, psychoanalysis was the treatment modality employed. Patient data was acquired from sessions conducted four to five times weekly. Third, their observations were made against the background of an emerging "ego psychology" where focus was shifting away from the earlier id psychology of Freud and toward the adaptive and defensive operations of the ego.

Adolph Stern

Adolph Stern (1938) was a New York analyst who first used the term "borderline" to describe a series of patients who failed to benefit from traditional psychoanalytic treatment. Stern believed that he had identified, in this group of patients, a disorder clearly distinct from schizophrenia and the neuroses.

Many of the clinical characteristics now thought to be central to an understanding of the borderline syndrome appeared in Stern's early writing. Among those were the following:

1. Highly vulnerable to narcissistic injury with extreme hypersensitivity and negative reaction to all but the most gentle of therapeutic interventions.
2. Idealization and devaluation of significant others, particularly of the analyst.
3. Feelings of insecurity and overwhelming anxiety in the face of traumatic stress.
4. A rigid personality and a tendency toward projective mechan-

isms in an effort to blame intrapsychic difficulties on external circumstances.

Stern imagined that the vulnerable position assumed by these patients relative to the analyst accounted for much of their difficulty in experiencing and working through their well-contained anger and hostility. The borderline patient tended to form a clinging and dependent relationship with the analyst. Based on these observations, Stern suggested a number of useful modifications to classical analytic technique.

Helene Deutsch

In 1942, Helene Deutsch expanded her earlier description of the "as if" patient. The material presented was strikingly similar to that discussed by Stern and served to carry the psychostructural understanding of the borderline patient another step forward. Deutsch characterized the "as if" patient as having a lack of self-identity that led to a personality style devoid of any constant features. The "as if" patient responded to the expectations of the environment in a chameleon-like way. The patient moved through life "as if" normal but lacked a real sense of self. Other features cited by Deutsch included a fully maintained grasp of reality, a masking of all aggressive tendencies, and a narcissistic identification with others in an attempt to remedy the inner sense of emptiness.

Deutsch was among the first clinicians to focus on the internal world of the borderline patient relative to pathological object relationships. She believed that in their pregenital development, these patients devalued the objects that could have served them as models for personality development, and thus failed to attain a sense of personal identity. Both Stern and Deutsch laid the groundwork for the development of later exploration into the pathological object relations, identity disturbance, primitive defense mechanisms, and affective instability of the borderline patient.

DESCRIPTIVE PSYCHOPATHOLOGY

The descriptive psychopathologists were concerned less with the intrapsychic and metapsychological workings of the mind and attended more to the behavioral criteria characteristic of the patient population being studied. Influenced strongly by Bleuler, these researchers believed that the so-called "borderline" patient of Stern and the "as if" patient of Deutsch were in fact subtypes of schizophrenia.

In 1941, Zilboorg introduced the term "ambulatory schizophrenia." Individuals with this diagnosis did not meet the strict Krapelinean definition of schizophrenia, did not need hospitalization, and maintained an adequate social facade. They nonetheless demonstrated clinical characteristics that suggested to Zilboorg a close relationship to schizophrenia. The ambulatory schizophrenic patient manifested oddities of thought, inability to sustain stable life pursuits, and characteristically unstable interpersonal relationships. Zilboorg believed that these patients as well as many of those in the analytic literature were in fact in the earliest stages of the schizophrenic process.

Hoch and Polatin (1949) further elaborated on the description of these patients when they described the "pseudoneurotic forms of schizophrenia." Like Zilboorg, Hoch and Polatin maintained that they were looking at a schizophrenic subtype in keeping with Bleuler's broad concept of the illness. Among the salient clinical features noted were diffuse free-floating anxiety, multiple neurotic symptoms, and diverse and perverse sexual practices.

Hoch and Polatin emphasized that "pseudoneurotic schizophrenia" was a "trait" diagnosis that was constant over time and not a transient "state." They held firm in maintaining that this was not a "borderline" group of patients but a genuine variant of schizophrenia.

ROBERT KNIGHT: THE FIRST SYNTHESIS

Between 1920 and 1950, many other works appeared describing patients who in one way or another shared similarities with the now-emerging "borderline patient." Marked polarity remained between the psychostructural thinking of the psychoanalytic movement and the descriptive entries of those more concerned with phenomenological criteria. It was not until Robert Knight's paper, "Borderline States" (1953), that some synthesis of these conceptual models was accomplished.

Knight combined the descriptive data and the psychostructural formulations that preceded him. He described an ego "state" which was called "borderline" and implied that the patient could enter into and emerge from this pathological condition. (This was in marked contrast to Kernberg's later concept of a fixed and immutable personality organization.)

Descriptively, Knight noted that these patients tended to manifest multiple neurotic symptoms. In keeping with the observations of Hoch and Polatin, Knight agreed that the clinical picture could be dominated by hysterical, phobic, obsessive-compulsive, and psychosomatic features.

Knight went beyond the descriptive psychopathology however and applied the concepts of psychoanalytic ego psychology. Having noted that these patients were "falling apart on the couch," Knight postulated that elements of ego weakness could account for this regressive tendency in the unstructured environment of psychoanalysis.

The ego weaknesses suggested by Knight were observed in what he called microscopic and macroscopic ways. Microscopic evidence of ego weakness was notable in the form of impaired integration of ideas, impaired judgment, thought blocking, peculiarities of word usage, and inappropriateness of affect. Macroscopic evidence was gleaned from a more distant view of the patient's functional level. Patients in the borderline state evidenced lack of concern over their life predicament, lack of achievement over time, unrealistic planning, and bizarre dreams.

Knight believed that the borderline state could be understood as being closely related to schizophrenia, as a time-limited condition, and as a reflection of definite though transient weaknesses in ego function.

PSYCHOSTRUCTURAL AND DESCRIPTIVE PSYCHOPATHOLOGY: LATER DEVELOPMENTS

Knight's synthesis of preceding attempts to understand and to describe the borderline patient set the stage for continued psychostructural and descriptive investigation. Otto Kernberg is representative of the psychostructural movement in the 1960s while the work of Roy Grinker clearly demonstrates the application of empirical research to the further development of a descriptive system of diagnosis.

Otto Kernberg

Influenced strongly by the work of Melanie Klein, Fairbairn, and Jacobson, Kernberg (1967, 1975) bases his understanding of the borderline patient in the framework of object relations theory. He defines object relations theory as the psychoanalytic approach to the internalization of interpersonal relations and postulates four stages through which the normal infant proceeds in developing an integrated mental representation of himself and of others. Kernberg's stages may be summarized as follows:

Stage 1. The first month of life, referred to as the stage of "normal autism" by Mahler (1979), antidates the establishment of an early, undifferentiated self-object (infant-mother) representation in the infant's mind.

Stage 2. During the second and third months of life, the infant imagines two internalized dyads to be coexistent. The first consists of the good self and the good mother while the second consists of the bad self and the bad mother. Pleasurable, gratifying experiences with mother are what constitute this mental image of a good self and good object while frustrating, ungratifying experiences make up the imagined bad self and bad mother unit. Still symbiotic with mother during this phase of development, the only differentiation that exists is between good and bad.

Stage 3. This stage marks the emerging intrapsychic differentiation of the infant from mother, of self from object. The infant begins to imagine himself as separate from mother within the good self-object representations. The good infant is now becoming a separate entity from the good mother. Later, this same separation of self from object will take place within the core "bad" representations. This stage occurs during the ninth through the twelfth month.

Stage 4. Kernberg's final developmental stage postulates the integration of good and bad self into the beginning of an integrated self-concept. The infant no longer experiences himself as all good or all bad but rather as a combination of good and bad feelings. Likewise, mother is not all gratifying nor is she all depriving; rather, she is an integration of both.

Kernberg imagines that an arrest at Stage 1 of these four stages of object relations development might yield a psychotic personality organization in which the individual is unable to distinguish between self and object, between inner reality and external reality. In much the same way, a borderline patient is imagined to be arrested at Stage 3. This results in a relatively sound ability to differentiate inner from outer reality but a failure to integrate "good" and "bad" mental representations of self and others. The infant as well as the outside world are experienced as all bad at one moment and as all good at another. No homogeneous blending of the two seems to take place.

The borderline patient is seen as having a fixed and stable ego structure reflected in this arrested development scheme. Unlike Robert Knight, who believed the borderline state was transient, Kernberg contends that the borderline personality organization is relatively constant.

Kernberg's theoretical construction of the borderline personality organization may be divided into three parts: (1) the descriptive features, (2) the structural analysis, and (3) the genetic-dynamic analysis. A brief review follows.

Kernberg agrees with those who preceded him in reporting that a multitude of neurotic symptoms are present in the borderline patient. Diffuse anxiety, phobias, obsessive-compulsive symptoms, and dissociative reactions may all be observed. In addition, a multitude of varying sexual deviations and "acting-out" behaviors are characteristic. These constitute the descriptive features.

The structural diagnosis is somewhat more complex but refers basically to those elements of the personality that are secondary to the infant's failure to integrate good and bad mental representations. The structural analysis considers three aspects of ego function: (1) reality testing, (2) identity, and (3) defense mechanisms.

Reality testing tends to be relatively well preserved in the borderline patient. While lapses in reality testing with short-lived psychotic episodes may be seen, this is not a pervasive state.

Identity diffusion is the term used by Kernberg to describe the patient's inability to formulate an integrated sense of self or others. The patient experiences himself one way at one moment and another way at a later point in time. Opposing images of the self coexist side by side with little appreciation of their contradictory relation. Similarly, objects in the outside world are experienced in equally discrepant terms. A spouse may be described to the therapist as warm, generous, and concerned. Shortly thereafter, that same spouse may be scorned as being cold, aloof, and indifferent. When confronted with this apparent contradiction, the patient only relates to the most immediate mental image of the spouse with little sense that the two descriptions are either contradictory or alternate sides of the same individual.

The primitive defense mechanisms noted by Kernberg all tend to function in the service of preserving the all-good and the all-bad view of the world. This is more broadly described by Schulz (1980), who considers the patient to function in an "all-or-none" mode.

Splitting is the primary defense characteristic of the borderline personality organization. The borderline patient sees the world as a series of all or none, black and white, encounters. Some people are good, others bad; no one is in between. It is not uncommon that a borderline inpatient will foster conflict among members of the treatment team by insisting that "some staff members understand me and care about me while others are hostile and malicious." If not recognized as a manifestation of the splitting operation, such polarization of the treatment team members will lead to internal strife and a sabotaging of the treatment plan.

Supporting the splitting operations of the ego are secondary defenses that reinforce the notion of the world as all one way or all another. Significant individuals are overvalued or devalued in what Kernberg calls "primitive idealization," "omnipotence," and "devaluation." "Denial by negation" is also employed to make the patient's emotions as well as the responses of others fit into a rigidly held image of the world. A patient will frequently dismiss an observation by the therapist as clearly misperceived and inaccurate. This negation of reality allows unacceptable impulses to be disowned and conflictual emotions dismissed as irrelevant or nonexistent.

Finally, Kernberg writes of "projective identification" as a hallmark defense. Objects, other people, are viewed by the patient as aggressive, while in fact, the patient is experiencing aggressive feelings himself that are projected onto the object. The borderline patient attempts to deal with the projected aggressive feelings in the other person as a first step toward dealing with the same feelings in himself. The patient who begins a session by commenting "It must take a lot of restraint on your part to see me for 50 minutes, as angry as I know you are with me," demonstrates the projected affect of hostility and the patient's identification with the therapist's imagined restraint in dealing with that hostility.

In discussing the genetic and dynamic features of the borderline patient, Kernberg elaborates extensively on pregenital and genital impulses. For purposes of this article, it can be stated that Kernberg views the borderline patient as fraught with feelings of aggression and rage that permeate all stages of psychosexual development.

Using Kernberg's thesis, the diagnosis of borderline personality organization is made when one sees a combination of highly suggestive signs and symptoms, good reality testing, identity diffusion, and a host of primitive defensive mechanisms. This constellation tends to be supported in turn by genetic and dynamic evidence for considerable aggression and oral rage permeating early stages of psychosexual development.

Roy Grinker

While Kernberg pursued an understanding of the borderline patient from the standpoint of object relations theory and impaired operations of the ego, Roy Grinker (1968) was more interested in the behavioral manifestations of the syndrome. Employing systematic, empirical research methodology, sophisticated statistical analyses, and a large patient population, Grinker designated four borderline subtypes based on readily observable behavioral manifestations of ego function.

Perry and Klerman (1978) summarized Grinker's findings and noted four common characteristics of all borderline patients as well as characteristics particular to each of the four individual subtypes.

Grinker's findings common to all borderline patients included anger as the primary affect, impaired interpersonal relationships, lack of consistent self-identity, and a pervasive depressive affect. The four borderline subtypes postulated by Grinker are the following:

Type 1: The Psychotic Border. Most closely related to the schizophrenic-like illnesses described by Zilboorg, Hoch, and Polatin, these patients behave inappropriately and unadaptively. They have a deficient sense of reality testing and self-identity. In addition to depression, major affective disturbances in the form of negativism and expressed anger are prominent.

Type 2: The Core Borderline Syndrome. These patients demonstrate chaotic interpersonal relationships, poor self-identity, depression, and a tendency to act out.

Type 3: The Adaptive "As If" Borderline. Resembling most closely the borderline of Stern and Deutsch, Grinker found these individuals to behave appropriately, engage in complementary relationships, demonstrate constricted affect with little spontaneity, and utilize a rigid intellectualized defensive posture.

Type 4: Border with Neurosis. This represents a somewhat healthier, more functional group of patients. Primary characteristics include a tendency toward depression, diffuse anxiety, and a multitude of neurotic and narcissistic features.

While Grinker did not go so far as to define clear inclusion and exclusion criteria for the diagnosis of the borderline patient, he attempted to objectify the diagnosis in a systematic manner, relying more heavily on observable behavior than on psychological inference. The pervasive presence of depression is of particular importance in Grinker's findings. This observation contributed to the later thinking that certain subtypes of the borderline syndrome may in fact be related genetically to the major affective disorders.

GUNDERSON AND SINGER: A SECOND SYNTHESIS

In much the same way that Robert Knight's paper synthesized the analytic and descriptive writings that preceded him, Gunderson and Singer distilled the work of Kernberg, Grinker, and others into a constellation of six clinical features considered central to the borderline disorder. Gunderson and Singer proposed the following diagnostic criteria:

1. Intense Affect: Depression and overt hostility were the most prominent of the affective symptoms displayed.
2. Impulsive Behavior: The borderline patient is prone to impulsive acting out that is ego-syntonic at the time of occurrence and ego-dystonic thereafter. Drug dependence, sexual acting out, and self-destruction behaviors are common.
3. Social Adaptiveness: Similar in nature to Deutsch's "as if" behaviors, this characteristic finding is manifested in appropriate social, academic, and occupational behavior derived more from mimicry and imitation than from an inner sense of personal identity.
4. Brief Psychotic Episodes: Frequently of a paranoid nature, these episodes are short lived and often precipitated by stress, drug use, and unstructured situations.
5. Interpersonal Relationships: Though relationships are general-

ly transient and superficial, the borderline patient will periodically enter into an intense, dependent relationship with much manipulation, demandingness, and devaluation.

6. Psychological Testing: Gunderson was among the first to consider the role of psychological testing in the diagnosis of the borderline patient. He noted adequate functioning on structured batteries with regression to bizarre, primitive responses to unstructured projective tests.

This work is particularly significant, as Perry and Klerman point out, not only because it served as a point of synthesis for earlier work but because it likewise was a base of departure from which more recent research would evolve.

RECENT DEVELOPMENTS—DONALD KLEIN, SEYMOUR KETY, ROBERT SPITZER

The family and genetic studies of Kety, Rosenthal, and Wender (1968) have contributed yet another perspective to attempts at sorting out the diagnostic complexities associated with the borderline concept. In examining the biological relatives of patients having been given a diagnosis of chronic schizophrenia, they made a particularly interesting observation. In addition to having an increased frequency of relatives who themselves warranted a diagnosis of chronic schizophrenia, these index cases also had an increased frequency of relatives who met the previously described criteria for ambulatory schizophrenia of Zilboorg and pseudoneurotic schizophrenia of Hoch and Polatin. These individuals, while not being actively psychotic, demonstrated oddities of thought, brief episodes of cognitive distortion, flattened affect, and a multitude of neurotic symptoms.

Concurrent with the work of Kety et al., was the ongoing research of Donald Klein. Klein and his colleagues had described a number of syndromes which they believed fell within the realm of affective disorder. They termed these "the phobic reaction," "the emotionally unstable character disorder," and "hysteroid-dysphoria." Klein believed that many of these syndromes overlapped with a number of borderline subtypes proposed by Grinker (Types 1, 2, and 4) as well as with many of the earlier descriptions of borderline patients. Klein's postulation that certain of the borderline syndromes may be related to the family of affective disorders is supported by studies reviewed in Stone's 1981 text.

The importance of these observations is that they again raise a very important question. Is it in fact possible, as speculated by early writers, that one group of patients whom we call borderline are genetically related to the schizophrenic disorders and that another group is a variant of affective illness? If this were the case, there would be profound implications for diagnosis, treatment, and prognosis.

Klein in his work with hysteroid-dysphoria has reported that a significant number of patients have responded favorably and specifically to MAO inhibitors. He asserts that most of these patients likewise meet the criteria for borderline disorder as set forth by Kernberg and Gunderson.

Spitzer (1979), in an attempt to incorporate the work of Kety and Klein into his research diagnostic criteria and later into DSM III, chose to consider the borderline patient as falling into one of two subtypes: (1) the schizotypal personality disorder; and (2) the unstable personality disorder. Each takes into account much of the earlier work reviewed in this article but also takes note of the familial and possibly genetic findings of Kety as well as the pharmacologic research of Klein.

For Spitzer, the schizotypal borderline personality disorder is more closely related to schizophrenia and is characterized by:

1. Odd communication though not grossly psychotic;
2. Ideas of reference;
3. Suspiciousness or paranoid ideation;
4. Recurrent illusions;
5. Magical thinking;
6. Poor rapport;
7. Social anxiety or hypersensitivity;
8. Social isolation

The unstable borderline personality, resembling the borderline patient of Kernberg and the hysteroid-dysphoric patient of Klien, is characterized by:

1. Identity disturbance;
2. Unstable and intense interpersonal relationships;
3. Impulsivity;
4. Inappropriate and intense anger;

5. Self-damaging acts;
6. Below-average work and school history;
7. Affective instability;
8. Chronic feelings of emptiness or boredom;
9. Problems tolerating being alone.

The borderline personality disorder in DSM III (1980) most resembles Spitzer's description of the unstable personality disorder. DSM III places little emphasis on psychostructural criteria. While incorporating many of the descriptive criteria noted by Kernberg, no attempt is made to include characteristic ego operations, particularly the primitive defense mechanisms. DSM III is a return to a phenomenologic or descriptive system of classification with attention away from intrapsychic or psychostructural phenomena.

The schizotypal personality disorder of DSM III tends to reflect more closely the schizophrenic end of the borderline continuum with diagnostic criteria derived from Spitzer's description of the schizotypal borderline patient.

It is important to note that DSM III is composed of descriptive criteria that do not rely on inference of intrapsychic processes to establish or exclude a given diagnosis. This system is not entirely compatible with the psychostructural notion of the borderline personality organization as advanced by Kernberg. In Kernberg's system of diagnosis, one may see a variety of personality disorders against a background of a borderline personality structure. Thus, it is important to clarify in one's mind a distinction between personality traits (such as, dependent, narcissistic, schizoid) and personality organization (neurotic, borderline, psychotic).

SUMMARY

An overview of the origin and evolution of the borderline concept has been presented. The early work of Kraepelin, Freud, and Bleuler were seen to lay the foundation for later systems of diagnosis and classification. The early metapsychologists, Stern, Deutsch, and others, provided insight into the psychological dynamics of the borderline patient and suspected that they were describing a disorder distinct from schizophrenia and the neuroses. Concurrently, early psychopathological descriptions, notably the work of Zilboorg, Hoch, and Polatin, contributed significantly to our phenomenological understanding of these patients whom they considered schizophrenic subtypes. Robert Knight in the early 1950s and John Gunderson in the mid-1970s synthesized the work that preceded them. Of the psychostructural writings on the borderline patient, Otto Kernberg was considered representative, while Roy Grinker's research epitomized a more empirical approach to the problem of diagnostic criteria. The impact of early family and genetic studies as well as the evolving body of pharmacological literature were considered relevant to the appreciation of our current system of diagnosis of the borderline personality disorder as detailed in DSM III.

While clear lines of delineation can never be presumed to exist in so complex a body of literature, this paper has demonstrated certain identifiable historical trends that may serve as a framework on which to base a more comprehensive study of the borderline concept.

REFERENCES

American Psychiatric Association. *Diagnostic and Statistical Manual of Mental Disorders (3rd Ed.)*, Washington, DC, 1980.

Bleuler, E. *Dementia Praecox or the Group of Schizophrenias*, NY: International Universities Press, 1950.

Capponi, A. Origin and evolution of the borderline patient. In: LeBoit, J. & Capponi, A., eds. *Advances in Psychotherapy of the Borderline Patient*, NY: Jason Aronson, 1979.

Deutsch, H. Some forms of emotional disturbance and their relationship to schizophrenia. *Psychoanalytic Quarterly*, 1942, *11*:301-321.

Freud, S. On beginning the treatment (further recommendations on the technique of psychoanalysis). (1913) In: Strachey, J., ed., *The Standard Edition of the Complete Psychological Works of Sigmund Freud, Vol. XII*, London: The Hogarth Press, 1961, pp. 123-144.

Grinker, R. R., Sr., Werble, B., & Drye, R. C. *The Borderline Syndrome*, NY: Basic Books, 1968.

Gunderson, J. G. & Singer, M. T. Defining borderline patients: An overview. *American Journal of Psychiatry*, 1975, *132*:1-10.

Hoch, P. H. & Polatin, P. Pseudoneurotic forms of schizophrenia. *Psychiatric Quarterly*, 1949, *23*:248-276.

Kernberg, O. F. Borderline personality organization. *Journal of the American Psychoanalytic Association*, 1967, *15*:641-685.

Kernberg, O. F. *Borderline Conditions and Pathological Narcissism*, NY: Jason Aronson, 1975.

Kety, S. S., Rosenthal, D., Wender, P. H., & Schulsinger, F. Mental illness in the biological and adoptive families of adopted schizophrenics. In: Rosenthal, D. & Kety, S. (eds.), *Transmission of Schizophrenia*, 1968, Oxford: Pergamon Press, pp. 345-362.

Klein, D. F., Gittelman, R., Quitkin, F., Rifkin, A. *Diagnosis and Drug Treatment of Psychiatric Disorders: Adults and Children*, Baltimore: Williams & Wilkins, 1980.

Knight, R. P. Borderline states. *Bulletin of the Menninger Clinic*, 1953, *17*:1-12.

Lehmann, H. E. Schizophrenia: Introduction and treatment. In: *Comprehensive Textbook of*

Psychiatry, Freedman, A. M., Kaplan, H. I., Sadock, B. J. (eds.), (2nd Ed.), 1975, Baltimore: Williams & Wilkins, pp. 851-859.

Mahler, M. S. *The Selected papers of Margaret S. Mahler*, Vol. I, NY: Jason Aronson, 1979.

Moore, B. E. & Fine, B. D. *A Glossary of Psychoanalytic Terms and Concepts*, 1967, NY: American Psychoanalytic Association.

Schulz, C. G. All-or-none phenomena in the psychotherapy of severe disorders. *The Psychotherapy of Schizophrenia*, edited by: John S. Strauss et al., Publisher: Plenum Publishing Corporation, NY, 1980.

Spitzer, R. L., Endicott, J. & Gibbon, M. Crossing the border into borderline personality and borderline schizophrenia. *Archives of General Psychiatry*, 1979, *36*:17-24.

Stern, A. Psychoanalytic investigation of and therapy in the borderline group of neuroses. *Psychoanalytic Quarterly*, 1938, *7*:467-489.

Stone, M. H. *The Borderline Syndromes, Constitution, Personality and Adaptation*, NY: McGraw-Hill, 1980.

Zilboorg, G. Ambulatory schizophrenias. *Psychiatry*, 1941, *4*:149-155.

Occupational Therapy Treatment: Interventions with Borderline Patients

Gail B. Goodman, OTR

ABSTRACT. This paper describes borderline phenomenon as it relates to occupational therapy treatment groups. The author discusses the genesis of the syndrome from the separation-individuation phase, its relation to adult functioning, subsequent treatment design and recommended therapeutic interventions. A case illustration will highlight these elements.

Developmental theory offers the occupational therapist a basis from which to understand human behavior. From infancy, the human being struggles to attain distinct milestones in several areas of functioning—perceptual-motor, cognitive, intellectual and emotional. An individual must move sequentially through various stages of development and fully integrate at each stage. A lack of completion at any stage will affect the individual's adaptive functioning. The borderline patient has not developed past the time of separation-individuation when the individual is utilizing the non-human environment as a projective recipient for conflicting emotional states. (Mahler, 1980; Rinsley, 1977; Searles, 1960) The particular phase of separation-individuation he finds difficult is rapprochement. The borderline patient has not attained the developmental milestones of internalized integration of opposing feeling states, nor a fully developed self-identity (Kernberg, 1975, 1980). Consequently, his experience of, and response to the external environment mirrors that of the toddler in rapprochement.

Gail B. Goodman is a private consultant.

TRANSITIONAL OBJECT PHENOMENON

The task of the toddler is to move from the earlier state of symbiosis to one of separation-individuation. Motorically, the child becomes able to move from mother by crawling, creeping and eventually walking. At the same time, he is learning that he is different from mother and begins to formulate a self-identity. Initial attempts at separating will induce anxiety until he has learned that even when separate, he is still "okay." The mother's role is to reward independent acts so that the child retains positive associations as he continues to explore the outside world. Should the mother continue to reward clinging, dependent and symbiotic behaviors rather than independent ones, the task of separation is thwarted (Abrams and Neubauer, 1978; Adler, 1975; Mahler, 1980; Rinsley, 1977). Fear of the loss of mothering and a heightened sense of anxiety cause the child to maintain a negative association with separation.

The child's efforts to develop a self-concept must be supported by a positive experience of separation. He uses the non-human environment to assist him in keeping positive feelings by attributing negative introjects to toys and other objects. He can then gain control over the feelings by controlling the objects. The non-human environment offers no resistance to the toddler (Barkin, 1978; Horner, 1979; McDevitt, 1980; Searles, 1960). The adult world of words, actions and emotions can be simplified by compartmentalization of good and bad into separate categories. The toddler experiences a greater sense of control over objects that do not talk back and punish. When attempts at ventilation of feelings become overwhelming, the child can resort to his easily manipulated non-human world.

It is at this time the child will attach himself to favored objects because he uses them as protective recipients for feeling states that are conflicting (Abrams and Neubauer, 1978; Searles, 1960). He will simplify his inner turmoil when confronted with the experience of "I'm bad" by projecting this onto his teddy bear so that he can regain the feeling state of "I'm good." It is a common sight to observe a young child scolding his toys with the same intonation used regarding his own behavior just moments before. He will also act out good feelings by cuddling his toys and cooing soothing words of affection. These favored toys have a special significance for the child. They are his shield and companion in rapprochement. Transitional objects are the toddler's "other half" until he has the capacity to integrate both good and bad introjects simultaneously. He will then relinquish these objects because he no longer needs to project various feeling states. He has a more integrated concept of himself as separate from mother.

The borderline patient does not fully succeed at this task of separation (Adler, 1975; Kernberg, 1980; Mahler, 1980; Masterson, 1975, 1976). Therefore, he maintains splitting as a major defense and externalizes his emotions in order to control them (Kernberg, 1975; Masterson, 1975). For the borderline patient, all the world is a potential transitional object. Objects in the life of the adult borderline patient suffer the same fate as earlier transitional objects (Arkema, 1981). A constant back and forth is experienced between the patient and his non-human world because he is in a chronic state of precarious balance between good and bad introjects (Adler, 1975; Masterson, 1976; McDevitt, 1980; Rinsley, 1977).

As with the object world, interpersonal relationships are colored by his lack of full individuation. There is a lack of clarity between the self and others. (Kernberg, 1975; Masterson, 1976) His perceptions of others become distorted by his vascillation between good and bad feeling states. He attributes his feelings to others and attempts to control his internal feeling states by attempting to control others (Adler, 1977; Kernberg, 1975).

If the non-human environment must be utilized as a projective recipient, the borderline cannot experience objects and activities as a source of pleasure (Arkema, 1981; Hartocollis, 1977; Kernberg, 1975). Had he continued along the developmental path, he would have moved toward a stage where the act of manipulating objects is enjoyable in its own right rather than as an emotional necessity. With a capacity for sublimation, a person can commit himself to an activity for its intrinsic enjoyment. True sublimation allows for an investment in the process itself, rather than its narcissistic rewards (Kernberg, 1975). The difference would be seen in the artist who derives enjoyment from the process of painting instead of being focused on finishing the painting because it will bring praise from others. For the borderline patient the canvas becomes a place to dump unpleasant feelings, and the end result may cause disgust and subsequent rejection. Or the painting, in being a projection of his poorly formulated self, takes on heightened meaning and requires approval from others.

Without the capacity to sublimate and enjoy the non-human world in a different context, all ordinary life tasks become difficult. Coupled with his confusion over interpersonal relationships, the borderline patient has a poor adaptation to society's demands and cannot feel success and satisfaction in both vocational and avocational pursuits (Hartocollis, 1977; Gunderson, 1977; Perry and Klerman, 1980).

Those concepts most germane to understand the treatment of borderline pathology are:

1. maintenance of splitting as a defense
2. use of the non-human environment, and
3. the lack of sublimation

THE DEVELOPMENT OF OCCUPATIONAL THERAPY GROUPS

The major modality of treatment used by the occupational therapist is the activity group, which meets the vocational, avocational and interpersonal needs of the patient. Depending upon the individual's level of cognitive skill, motor coordination and interpersonal adeptness, task-oriented groups of various levels are implemented. The goal is to improve the patient's functional adaptation. Discussion is an adjunct to the activity in order to foster improved self-awareness of the intrapsychic issues underlying the process of the task and the patient's response to it. Depending upon the patient's particular pathology, the approach may be either supportive or confronting. In designing a treatment group for a specific population, the therapist evaluates the following criteria:

a. the goal of the group
b. the target population
c. the modalities used
d. the role of the therapist
e. the frequency and duration of the group

The goal of work groups is to adjust the patient's activity style in the context of an employment setting. A person's functioning at work is dependent upon his capacity to understand what is expected of him and to carry out the task. Simultaneously, he must become part of a cooperative group whereby interpersonal relationships are developed for the purpose of producing a mutually agreed upon outcome. Appropriate relationships must be established with authority figures (i.e., bosses and supervisors) and peers (i.e., co-workers). Occupational therapy work adjustment groups should be set up as realistically as possible so that they may be a practice ground. Groups that use a model of supervisors, co-workers, deadlines and specific assignments are effective. When problems with performance arise, the discussion should focus on why the group or individual cannot meet agreed upon expectations.

The borderline patient's problems in functioning at work fall into the areas of interpersonal relationships and an incapacity to separate the task from his intrapsychic imbalance between feeling good and feeling bad. The work environment becomes fused with his struggle to maintain a self-concept that is separate from those with whom he interacts (Adler, 1975; Gunderson, 1977; Masterson, 1976). He will be a difficult employee because criticism and praise will mirror his dependent vs. independent issues. With supervisors, he will exhibit alternating behaviors that re-enact the rapprochement he has failed to complete. Although his cognitive abilities to understand instructions are usually unaffected by his psychopathology, he often cannot perform the task without re-experiencing the earlier need to project onto non-human objects (Arkema, 1981). He will be unable to just "do what is expected" without attaching inappropriate significance to the whole experience. Intolerance for anxiety and a propensity for impulsive behavior (Carpenter, Gunderson and Strauss, 1977; Kernberg, 1975; Masterson, 1976) may lead to sudden resignations and/or inappropriate acting-out on the job. The satisfactions available to others will be impossible for the borderline patient (Hartocollis, 1977; Masterson, 1976; Perry and Klerman, 1980).

The borderline patient's inability to sublimate (Kernberg, 1975) is seen in a history of unsatisfactory leisure-time experiences and a lack of involvement in activities that enhance a sense of well-being. The occupational therapist will prescribe a recreational activity, either individual or group, knowing that it will re-create these difficulties. The goal of leisure groups is to help the patient recognize his problems within the non-work environment and adjust dysfunctional patterns. Again, the problematic arenas are the patient's relationship with the human and non-human stimuli within social contexts. In choosing an activity, he will re-experience his dilemma with the non-human environment and its subsequent significance. The mere act of selecting an activity that can be enjoyable is difficult because he does not perceive activities as a source of satisfaction.

This is part of the treatment process. The patient's execution of a task, once selected, will exacerbate his inability to enjoy doing and might be distinctly unpleasant. The therapist must understand the underlying process that is obstructing the patient's capacity to experience pleasure.

Creative-expressive media provide a unique outlet for individuals who are struggling with intangible unconscious issues. The creative process facilitates the merging of one's self with the creation, (Kris, 1952) thereby encouraging projection. Art can be self-reflective; it can be a source of insightful discussion. The therapist's role in creative groups is to keep control over the process through selection of media, observation of the patient and timely interventions.

Case Illustration

The following case illustration will be used to highlight the functional difficulties experienced by the borderline patient.

Cheryl is a 27-year-old divorced white female. The primary complaint upon admission was chronic amphetamine abuse for four years, coupled with an inability to organize her life activities; an inconsistent work history and chaotic interpersonal relationships.

The patient's functioning was initially disrupted following her father's sudden death when she was thirteen, and then again at age fifteen when her mother remarried. The patient began to lose interest in school and run around with a "wild crowd." Her mother insisted she begin therapy. Despite her perception of the therapist as moralistic and judgmental, she remained in treatment for two years. At age seventeen, her anti-social behavior escalated—she indulged in multi-drug abuse and frequently ran away from home. On one such occasion, she was returned to her parents by a private detective they had hired. At nineteen, she attended college, changing schools and her course of study each year. Cheryl married in the beginning of college and then divorced during her senior year, expressing a fear of "being trapped in a boring life style." She stopped attending classes and began amphetamine abuse (both orally and intravenously). She never graduated from college. For a year, she was unable to attain employment and maintained a high level of drug use.

She then returned to her home town and tried to improve her situation. She resumed therapy, moved into her own apartment and got a job as a buyer for a department store. This period represents her most consistent employment situation. Despite her ability to maintain this job for two years, her social functioning continued to be chaotic. She was involved in a mutually abusive relationship with a woman and continued to use quaaludes and cocaine. She could not manage her money, often spending it excessively. She would appeal to her parents for funds but simultaneously complained about their intrusiveness. When she ended her job as a buyer, she opened up a small boutique. This lasted a brief time. She took a public relations job in a friend's club, taught scuba diving and returned to college for less than a semester. Each of these efforts represented a desperate attempt to do something meaningful and gratifying.

She went on a starvation diet and dropped her weight to 74 pounds in order to model for a friend who was a male homosexual hairdresser. She moved in with him. Their relationship was marked by sexual adventures with both men and women. Cheryl continued to use amphetamines to keep her weight down. Following a bizarre weekend orgy with her roommate, another male homosexual and a lesbian, she returned to her home town, locked herself in a hotel room and called her former therapist. He recommended long-term, in-hospital treatment. After a three-week diagnostic assessment, she was referred to a treatment unit for borderline patients.

Cheryl's involvement in occupational therapy will be used to illustrate how the borderline patient behaves in occupational therapy treatment groups. Specific interventions will be cited to exemplify the therapist's role and clarify how these interventions facilitate improved functioning.

THE TREATMENT PROCESS

Cheryl's treatment included participation in leisure groups that allowed for individual choice of activity. The first problem arose when she got caught in her own indecision about what to do. As with many borderline patients, she would have balked at any suggestions made (and, indeed, she did reject some ideas from staff) but she also experienced any lack of guidance as anxiety-inducing. The commitment to a task, above and beyond the narcissistic gains, was problematic. She sought the therapist's approval for her ideas and when most suggestions were greeted with equal acceptance, she floundered. Admittedly, the therapist was impressed with her idea of building a marionette and this may have influenced her final decision to tackle this project. Without any plan to follow, she secured herself extra time with the therapist to problem-solve the construction of the puppet.

The marionette was to be a female character. Its symbolic significance was apparent at the outset. Building the puppet became a re-enactment of the patient's struggle with her self-identity which was not fully integrated. Over the time she worked on it, the doll's identity changed from various tragic ballet heroines to literary figures such as Pinocchio (an androgynous character). She constantly sought approval over its construction, claiming its relation to the final outcome was important. She had difficulty deciding on the best technique for reinforcement of the limbs, taking excessive time to decide the position of the legs. It was apparent that her indecision was related to her confusion about the marionette's gender. After completing the torso and extremities, she became anxious over the size, shape and construction of the head. However, before she ever began work on the head, she cut off the arms. This incident was remarkable because Cheryl had a strong reaction to her destructiveness and it opened up a discussion of feelings. She simultaneously experienced depression and hatred; she laughed and cried. As she talked, she tried to defend against her feelings by claiming she had no reason to feel hate. The therapist confronted this as a rationalization and a defense against the feelings. The therapist's goal in the confrontation was to assist the patient in staying with the feelings, rather than allowing an intellectualization to take over (Masterson, 1976). Following this, Cheryl discussed having sensations of not being real. In her diffused self-concept, she could not get a grip on "the real Cheryl." Pointing out that her present feelings were real brought on a new onslaught of tears. She became frightened at the strength of her emotions and expressed a concern over hurting others with her feelings. She was given reassurance that her feelings could not harm others. The reality of her current feeling state was reiterated. She became silent for a while but then returned to her project. At the end of the session, she claimed to have enjoyed the work accomplished at the end of the treatment hour and took the puppet back to the unit to continue working on it.

The role of the occupational therapist was to assist the patient in recognizing unconscious feelings that were provoked. Secondly, the therapist worked for the maintenance of those feelings through a confrontation of the defenses. Thirdly, the patient was redirected towards the activity as an outlet for these feelings and a resolution of the inner conflict (Masterson, 1976). The recognition of feeling states is a stepping stone and it is the continuation of an activity that will promote improved functioning. There must be a marriage of discussion and doing.

The creative-expressive group can also be used to help borderline patients to integrate various feeling states. Prior to a long holiday weekend, the therapist conducted an art mural session. The mural group was used as a time to explore the patient's expectations; a subsequent meeting was used to plan activities.

As they drew, the patients laughed and joked, but upon seating themselves they saw that they had depicted groups of isolated people. There was a lack of community feeling amongst the people in the picture. The group became depressed and had difficulty in accepting the therapist's observation of their previous behavior. They were unable to integrate opposing feeling states, though closely connected by time. Although the group ended on a depressed note, the follow-up session to plan activities focused on resolution of the feared isolation through designated times for patients to interact. The therapist helped the group to improve a potentially negative experience (i.e., a long, lonely weekend) by offering adaptive alternatives.

Complementary activities, such as a mural followed by a community planning group, are jointly therapeutic. The therapist can assist patients in utilizing activities as a source of resolution for uncomfortable feelings.

When participating in a leisure-oriented or creative-expressive group, selection of an activity will be part of the treatment process and this initial commitment will be difficult, as exemplified by Cheryl's hesitation before deciding on a marionette. Choosing an activity for enjoyment requires a capacity to formulate an opinion on what will enhance self-pleasure. There must be a firm concept of the "I" experience before being able to state "I want to do that." Secondly, the activity must be seen as neutral territory which the act of doing will then alter (i.e., "This pile of clay will become a vase because I will change it.'') And finally, the mastery of skill required to manipulate objects into a desired end product must be perceived as rewarding, pleasurable and self-actualizing. All these possibilities are unavailable to the borderline patient (Searles, 1975). Once involved in the activity, the project will be subject to projection of the patient's vacillating feeling states. It will be alternately perceived as rewarding or disgusting (Arkema, 1981). Projects that end up in the garbage are grist for the therapeutic mill. They are concrete examples of projected feeling states. To promote resolution of these feelings they must first be recognized, and an investment in completion of the project must be encouraged.

A work adjustment group uses the cooperative group format. Group members must make decisions, accept group decisions, place expectations on each other and execute individual tasks. If the group is structured to allow for patient-to-patient feedback, the acting supervisor can discuss another patient's performance. In a newspaper group, for example, this could take the form of questioning incomplete assignments, facilitating a group decision or rejecting incorrect work. The therapist, if not performing the role of supervisor, must monitor the supervisor's style and, if necessary, set limits on overzealous patient supervisors. Verbal content and style are significant in a work environment. Inappropriate use of a supervisor's power should be discussed.

When participating in a vocational group, the borderline patient will re-experience past failures. His external behavior may vascillate between adamant refusal to accept assigned tasks and an overinvolvement in the assignment. When criticized, he will counteract with anger at the source of criticism. He will devalue the task or the entire project (Arkema, 1981). Others will be blamed for his incapacities and astute rationalizations will defend his perceptions. If he does not react with stony devaluation, he may become overwhelmingly depressed at his failure and take a masochistic position regarding his ineptness.

What is the underlying process of this behavior? The borderline patient does not have an integrated self-concept and is dependent upon others for positive associations with independent acts. Those who offer criticism are reminders of the rejecting experiences that were once part of his feeble attempts at separation. He will employ the defenses of splitting and projective identification as a way of avoiding a negative experience (Kernberg, 1975). Those interventions previously described can be used in vocational groups. The therapist clarifies the process and confronts the patient's defensive posture. Once the patient acknowledges his failure to perform the task as required, he will experience depression. At this point, the therapist should be aware of the need for the patient to remain with that feeling (Masterson, 1976). While recognizing that this is difficult, she should continue to support the group expectation that individuals perform as assigned. In the face of hostility or masochistic brow-beating, she should 1) confront the defensive style, 2) acknowledge the difficulty in accepting the underlying emotion, and 3) redirect the patient to the realities of the task. Resolution lies in the patient's ultimate capacity to experience various feelings but continue to perform (Adler, 1975; Masterson, 1976).

In vocational groups, task completion is important because it is a reality-based expectation. Employers have performance requirements that must be met. For vocational success an individual must ultimately do what he is told, not show insight as to why he is unable. The borderline patient who has a history of job failures will not benefit from excessive verbalizations on why he has not completed his assignments. Intellectualizations are a continuation of his denial (Kernberg, 1975). Eventually, he must face the issue by doing the work.

Much like a juggler, the therapist must keep the group's attention on the task while discussing difficulties that arise for individuals and the group as a whole. There is no formula for how much discussion is therapeutic and when a group has passed over the line into avoidance techniques. Verbalizations can improve understanding of vital issues but the occupational therapist knows that dysfunctional patterns are improved through the act of doing. Investment must be made in those behaviors that reflect internalization of the desired changes.

COUNTERTRANSFERENCE

Countertransferential issues can interfere with the therapist's capacity to maintain her objectivity. In his vascillation between angry devaluation and depressed emptiness, the borderline patient can induce strong feelings in the therapist (Adler, 1975; Masterson, 1976). It is likely that the therapist will become entangled in countertransferential feelings.

It is the role of the occupational therapist to focus on the function-

ing. She should not get involved in the "interpersonal-object relations—you vs. me" issues. Interpersonal issues will arise, but *they
should be dealt with in the context of the goals of the group.* The occupational therapist can utilize other team members to help keep a
handle on her countertransferential reactions (Adler, 1977). Without this type of support from the treatment team, the therapist can
lose sight of her role and objectivity. In order to intervene during a
group process, she must be able to separate out issues that are personal from those that are an outcome of her professional observations.

SUMMARY

Different occupational therapy treatment groups, whether they be
vocational, avocational or self-expressive, offer a specialized milieu
for the borderline patient. The therapist, in understanding the developmental milestones that have not been attained, can prescribe activities which facilitate re-enactment, discussion and resolution of
these issues. The patient brings his particular internal conflicts to the
treatment process and his external behaviors reflect those problems.
Treatment interventions should be:

1. observation and clarification of the underlying process
2. confrontation of the defensive behaviors
3. acknowledgement of provoked feeling states, and
4. redirection of the behaviors toward functional adaptations.

By designing treatment groups that allow for this type of intervention, the occupational therapist can help the borderline patient to improve his functional capacities.

REFERENCES

Abrams, S. & Neubauer, P.B. Transitional Objects: Animate and Inanimate. In S.A. Grol-
nick & L. Barkin (Eds.), *Between Reality and Fantasy—Transitional Objects and
Phenomena.* New York: Jason Aronson, Inc., 1978.
Adler, G. The Usefulness of the "Borderline" Concept in Psychotherapy. In J.E. Mack
(Ed.), *Borderline States in Psychiatry.* New York. Grune and Stratton, Inc., 1975.
Adler, G. Hospital Management of Borderline Patients and Its Relation to Psychotherapy. In
P. Hartocollis (Ed.), *Borderline Personality Disorders,* New York: International Univer-
sities Press, Inc., 1977.
Arkema, P.H. The Borderline Personality and Transitional Relatedness. *American Journal
of Psychiatry,* 1981, *138,* 172-177.

Barkin, L. The Concept of the Transitional Object. In S.A. Grolnick & L. Barkin (Eds.), *Between Reality and Fantasy—Transitional Objects and Phenomena*, New York: Jason Aronson, Inc., 1978.

Carpenter, W., Jr., Gunderson, J., & Strauss, J.S. Considerations of the Borderline Syndrome: A Longitudinal Comparative Study of Borderline and Schizophrenic Patients: In P. Hartocollis (Ed.), *Borderline Personality Disorders*, New York: International Universities Press, Inc., 1977.

Gunderson, J.G. Characteristics of Borderlines. In P. Hartocollis (Ed.), *Borderline Personality Disorders*, New York: International Universities Press, Inc., 1977.

Hartocollis, P. Affects in Borderline Disorders. In P. Hartocollis (Ed.), *Borderline Personality Disorders*, New York: International Universities Press, Inc., 1977.

Horner, A.J. *Object Relations and the Developing Ego in Therapy.* New York: Jason Aronson, Inc., 1979.

Kernberg, O.F. *Borderline Conditions and Pathological Narcissism.* New York: Jason Aronson, Inc., 1975.

Kernberg, O.F. Developmental Theory, Structural Organization and Psychoanalytic Technique. In R. Lax, S. Bach, & J.A. Burland (Eds.), *Rapprochement—The Critical Subphase of Separation-Individuation*, New York: Jason Aronson, Inc., 1980.

Kris, E. *Psychoanalytic Explorations in Art.* New York: International Universities Press, Inc., 1952.

Mack, J.E. *Borderline States in Psychiatry.* New York: Grune & Stratton, Inc., 1975.

Mahler, S. Rapprochement Subphase of the Separation-Individuation Process. In R.F. Lax, S. Bach, & J.A. Burland (Eds.), *Rapprochement—The Critical Subphase of Separation-Individuation*, New York: Jason Aronson, Inc., 1980.

Masterson, J.F. Intensive Psychotherapy of the Adolescent with a Borderline Syndrome. In G. Caplan (Ed.), *American Handbook of Psychiatry* (2nd ed.) New York: Basic Books, Inc., 1974.

Masterson, J.F. *Psychotherapy of the Borderline Adult—A Developmental Approach.* New York: Brunner/Mazel, Inc., 1976.

Masterson, J.F. The Splitting Defense Mechanism of the Borderline Adolescent: Developmental and Clinical Aspects. In J. Mack (Ed.), *Borderline States in Psychiatry,* New York: Grune & Stratton, Inc., 1975.

McDevitt, J.B. The Role of Internalization in the Development of Object Relations During the Separation-Individuation Phase. In R. Lax, S. Bach & J.A. Burland (Eds.), *Rapprochement—The Critical Subphase of Separation-Individuation*, New York: Jason Aronson, Inc., 1980.

Perry, J. & Klerman, G.L. Clinical Features of the Borderline Personality Disorder. *American Journal of Psychiatry,* 1980, *137,* 165-173.

Rinsley, D.B. An Object Relations View of Borderline Personality. In P. Hartocollis (Ed.), *Borderline Personality Disorders*, New York: International Universities Press, Inc., 1977.

Searles, H.F. *The Non-Human Environment—In Normal Development and Schizophrenia.* New York: International Universities Press, 1960.

Searles, H.F. Dual and Multiple Identity Processes in Borderline Ego Functioning. In P. Hartocollis (Ed.), *Borderline Personality Disorders*, New York: International Universities Press, Inc., 1977.

A Theoretical Approach
to the Treatment of Work Difficulties
in Borderline Personalities

Cheryl Salz, OTR

ABSTRACT. This paper reviews the psychodynamic basis of borderline personality disorder with special reference to work difficulties. The model of human occupation is reviewed, and its use as a theoretical framework for a formulation of borderline occupational functioning is proposed. A hypothetical model is conceptualized and the expected deficits in the volitional, habituation, and performance subsystems described. The primary occupational dysfunction of the borderline patient is shown to occur at the level of exploratory behavior, or play, and to manifest itself in the inability to perform autonomous adult roles. A treatment approach derived from this formulation is delineated, emphasizing the need for a context of exploration and curiosity. A specific treatment program is described and the therapeutic change process is illustrated through clinical case examples.

Jean ran a Karate school for ten years and has worked as an administrative assistant. She has not worked regularly in five years. She has made two serious suicide attempts and often reacts to pressure by cutting her arm with a razor blade. Don has been going to an Ivy League College for the last eight years, getting As and Bs when he doesn't drop out before the semester's end, and go on a wild drinking binge. Carol has performed musically with great success, has directed a theater, and can type 85 words a minute. She has been unable to work in three years and has a severe eating disorder characterized by binging and vomiting. These are brief profiles of

Cheryl Salz is an Occupational Therapy Supervisor, St. Lukes-Roosevelt Hospital, New York, NY.

A version of this paper was originally presented at the 1983 National Occupational Therapy Conference in Portland, Oregon under the title *A Comprehensive Activity Program for Borderline Patients.*

some of the borderline patients who attended activity and pre-vocational groups at the St. Luke's Acute Day Treatment Program over the last year. Despite excellent skills and impressive records of accomplishment, all had been painfully unable to maintain productive lifestyles. They were referred to day treatment by their primary therapists as a transition from hospitalization, or prolonged marginal functioning, to independent living.

The day treatment program provides a six to eighteen month rehabilitation program for borderline patients. It is located in Manhattan and employs four full-time clinical staff to serve a maximum of 28 patients. The typical patient is white, female, between 20 and 45 years old, well educated, and from an upper middle class family. The treatment model is a psychodynamically oriented therapeutic community. Two occupational therapists and a dance therapist were charged with developing activity approaches which would address the vocational, leisure, and expressive-creative needs of this population. While this paper suggests a general approach to borderline occupational functioning, the specific focus will be the development of an activity program designed to improve vocational functioning and facilitate return to work or school, a primary stated goal of most program members.

The vocational histories of these patients revealed serious functional deficits. Foremost among these was inconsistency, a work-school pattern characterized by intense involvement followed by abrupt, premature termination, often at the brink of success. Other common problems included: troubled, angry relationships with bosses and co-workers, lack of satisfaction derived from work, avoidance, procrastination, poor work habits, and unrealistically high expectations for perfection. In general, they hated work, felt hopeless about their ability to do it, were resistant to vocational activities, and frightened about their futures. They derived little pleasure from their considerable skills, and clung tenaciously to grandiose fantasies.

To develop a viable activity approach, the specific nature of borderline pathology was explored. The considerable literature on borderline personality has been contributed largely by psychoanalytically oriented clinicians. While this establishes diagnostic criteria and details for the psychodynamic basis for treating patients, the implications for direct activity intervention have not been well elaborated. The model of human occupation developed by Kielhofner and Burke (1980) was adopted as a framework for assessing and treating borderline occupational dysfunction. This paper shall review the developmental/psychodynamic formulation of the borderline syndrome, with special reference to work difficulties; assess the implications of this formulation for occupational behavior functioning; and suggest specific treatment approaches.

REVIEW OF THE LITERATURE

While there are many methods of categorizing borderline pathology, and differences of opinion about symptomatology, there is widespread agreement that the syndrome has its genesis in a failure of the mother-child interaction during the period Mahler (1975) identifies as the rapprochement subphase of separation-individuation (16-24 months). At this time the child begins to feel a sense of his separateness and struggles to become autonomous (colloquially called the "terrible twos"). During this phase the child's urge toward independence is insistent but fragile, and his feelings of dependence on the mother are intense and painful. He has become separate enough to realize the extent of his vulnerability. If the mother maintains a concerned interest in the child, and supports his independent exploration, he gradually develops an integrated internal sense of a competent, though limited self, and a separate but nurturing mother. If, however, the mother's need to maintain a dependent attachment between herself and her child is very strong, a different pattern develops. The mother may reward the child's dependent and clinging behavior, and reject efforts at autonomy (Rinsley, 1977); or she may withdraw, leaving the child genuinely alone and vulnerable (Mahler, 1975). Some theorists (Kernberg cited in Sass, 1982; Stern, 1977) have noted that constitutional features of the child, such as high activity level, excessive aggression, or difficulty processing arousal can contribute to a failure in the mother-child interaction. In any case, the separation-individuation process is not completed, and the child's developing sense of self is thwarted.

Many of the theorists who have looked at this phenomenon have identified a splitting or fragmenting of experience as a result. Kernberg (1975) views splitting as the underlying defense mechanism utilized by the borderline patient. In the normal individual, splitting occurs only during a brief developmental phase. The child's first internalized images of herself and of the mother, occurring under the aegis of strong positive and negative affects, are split into a good mother and good self image associated with positive experiences, and a bad mother and bad self image associated with negative experiences. The split images soon become integrated into a realistic image of the self and a realistic image of the mother. In the case of the borderline, the mother-child interaction is so unsatisfying that the bad tends to overwhelm the good, amounting to the loss of the loving mother. The child maintains split internalized images in order to preserve the pleasurable feeling of connection to the mother in the face of tremendous rage and frustration. The result is a rapid vacillation of contradictory states, without the stable and nourishing experience of relatedness which emerges from realistic, integrated images of the self and others. The polarities of good and bad do not allow for the experiencing of the myriad traits that make each individual unique, resulting in identity diffusion. Splitting also inhibits the neutralization of aggressive feelings which would allow them to be used for growth. Instead rage is acted out destructively. Libidinal object constancy, the ability to derive gratification by evoking the memory of a loved person is impaired, leading to the need for immediate gratification and difficulty in being alone. Additional ramifications of such a pattern include grandiosity and omnipotence (associated with the all good), and devaluation and denial (associated with the all bad).

Kernberg (1975) outlines a treatment approach involving verbal exploration, confrontation, and limit setting to help the patient become aware of and change these patterns as they manifest themselves in the therapeutic relationship. In the context of work issues, Kernberg's approach is useful in helping patients explore their erratic and impulsive work patterns, and in confronting the splitting which contributes to grandiose or devalued work fantasies. His techniques are useful in confronting distorted relationships with peers and bosses as they emerge in the context of activity groups. His work, however, does not lead to the heart of the issue of productivity.

Winnicott (1960) also concludes that there is a split which originates with the failed mother-child relationship. His concept is of a true and false self. Sutherland (1980) describes Winnicott's position beautifully:

> The fit between the baby's experience and the mother's response give the former an omnipotent, creative quality.

Repeated experiences of this kind establish in the infant a sense of wholeness, conviction about the goodness of reality, and a "belief in" the world as a rewarding place. This core of feeling gives rise to a "true self," because the full maturational potential, as it emerges in its increasing repertoire of activity, can be actualized in joyful relations. (pp. 833-834)

With increasing confidence the child is able to relinquish omnipotence for the pleasure and pains of genuine self expression and interaction. When the mother impinges too severely on the child's spontaneous expressions, this "true self" can not evolve. Rather, a "false self" forms which merely complies with the mother's expectations. The "false self" shields the "true self" which retreats from reality and is preserved as infantile omnipotence.

Fast (1975) reports a variant of the "true self"/"false self" split in her observations of the work difficulties of adults with borderline personality disorders. She identifies a bipartate work pattern in which work is experienced as meaningless, and engagement in it is undertaken in a deadened robotlike conformity without self involvement. Simultaneously, however, such persons often experience great enthusiasms, usually of a creative or artistic sort. She hypothesizes that there is no integration of pleasure and unpleasure in activity. Rather, creative activity is identified with the narcissistic pleasure world (the omnipotent or grandiose self) and purposeful action with unpleasure.

Winnicott (1971) identifies play as the universal facilitator for growth and feels that mutual playing is the essence of the psychotherapeutic relationship. He believes that it is only in playing that the individual uses his whole personality in creative activity, and it is only through creativity that one discovers the self. He implies an interactive system as a context for development, typified by his statement, "There is no such thing as a baby, there are only babies and mothers" (1960, p. 39). Neither he nor Fast, however, examine the mechanisms through which spontaneous play is shaped into adult productivity. They fail to delineate how the "false self" child becomes an adult with work difficulties.

The model of human occupation (Kielhofner and Burke, 1980) describes the dynamic process through which a person develops a capacity for meaningful, competent, purposeful activity. It can be useful in understanding the borderline's deficits in this area. Human occupation is presented as an open system. Individuals receive information from the environment (input). As this information interacts with internal mechanisms, strategies of response are developed (throughput) which lead to action (output). Information about the results of this action re-enters the system (feedback). The driving force of the system is conceptualized as the innate tendency toward mastery. Out of this global tendency, through dynamic interactions with the environment over time, a hierarchy of three differentiated subsystems evolves. The most basic of these, governing change in the others, is the volitional subsystem. It is composed of motivational structures: interest, valued goals, and personal causation (a sense of your self being the director of your action). Kielhofner[1] notes that it is not a motivational force in the traditional sense, it is more like the following collection of emotions: morale, joie de vivre, persistence, courage, and commitment. It is the drive civilized within the emotional and meaning framework of the culture. As the person matures, the level of enactment in this subsystem moves along a continuum from exploration (pre-school) to skill competency (grade school) to role achievement (adolescence). The habituation subsystem consists of internalized roles and habits, and serves to maintain patterns of behavior. The performance subsystem consists of skills and skill components. The system both changes and is changed by the environment in cycles of interaction. Those which support adaptation by rewarding competence and enhancing the individual's efficacy are benign cycles. Those in which output is consistently ineffective or unreinforced, lead to an expectation of failure and even less effective functioning, and are vicious cycles.

A MODEL OF BORDERLINE
OCCUPATIONAL FUNCTIONING

A hypothetical model of borderline occupational functioning was conceptualized using Kielhofner and Burke's formulation. Borderline pathology has its genesis in the period between 16 and 24 months (Mahler, 1975). At this point the playful, exploratory capacities of the child are greatly enhanced by the ability to walk, the development of fine motor coordination, and more sophisticated cognitive structures. The child can begin to assert his autonomy with an insistent ''no'' to parental demands. The parental response to these new functions plays a critical shaping role. An effective volitional subsystem, conceptually similar to Winnicott's ''true self,'' can only evolve in the context of a successful parent-child interaction. Kielhofner states in this regard:[1]

> Child's play is a behavior that requires the tutorship and caretaking of an adult. Without it the child, driven by a system that demands action, continues to act, but this action is not integrated into the sociocultural fabric. The child learns to imitate or please the mother, but does not experience play and work as emerging from the self.

Thus, the mother's thwarting of exploration in the case of the borderline patient, functions as a negatively reinforcing environment. There is no safe arena for exploratory play. A vicious cycle is set up leading to a defective volitional subsystem, or "false self." Winnicott and Kielhofner seem to be in complete agreement. The volitional system will be characterized by a split. Spontaneous goal directed activity emerging from the child's joy of exploration will be gradually devalued or disappear, the only pleasurable remnants remaining safely in fantasy. On the other hand, a great value will be placed on satisfying the demands of the mother, with activity directed only to that end, with no intrinsic enjoyment or feeling of self expression.

It is in understanding how this early childhood situation becomes manifested as the borderline syndrome in the adult that the occupational behavior model is most useful. The internalized roles remain fragmented and childlike: either a helpless child needing parental care, or a fragile, incompetent loner. While there is no realistically competent "doing," there is often a fantasized role of a grandiose "being" self: an *Artist*, a *Dancer*, etc. Habit patterns are severely impaired. Unfueled by the developing values and interests of the volitional system, patterns of response become limited and rigid, problem solving skills are poor, and there is little internal ability to modulate levels of stimulation. The performance subsystem includes predominantly those skills demanded by the mother or, later, the teacher. They may be practiced prodigiously and perfected, again with little inner feeling, except to the extent that the particular skill gratifies a grandiose fantasy.

The irony of this particular pattern of subsystem dysfunction is that as long as the mother and the environment remain consistent, the child's functioning appears fairly normal and well adapted. The child takes cues from the mother or teacher and the "false self" adequately fulfills the demands. Warning signals such as overinvolvement in fantasy, outbursts of rage, and general unhappiness are often overlooked because "the child is functioning" or "she's doing well in school." It is only during adolescence, when volitional enactment moves from skill competency to role achievement, that the deficit becomes glaringly apparent. The achievement of adult roles requires a level of autonomy the borderline has not obtained. As the adolescent moves from the structure of home and school, and can no longer rely on environmental cues, habituation deficits become obvious. With few exploratory strategies, responses become extremely impulsive and erratic. These impulsive patterns, combined with childlike internal roles, produce the chaotic and avoidant patterns of behavior so typical of borderline patients. Meaningless skills cannot now be incorporated into meaningful roles, and the sense of emptiness and futility becomes unbearable. Rather than assuming an autonomous role, the borderline continually seeks another person to depend on or rebel against. The struggle of childhood is continually repeated, and failure at adult social and vocational roles becomes more and more entrenched.

The preceding discussion is a hypothetical model of borderline functioning. Salz and White[2] are currently engaged in reviewing and developing evaluation tools to establish an empirical base for the model. In one preliminary study five patients were assessed using the *Survey of Study Habits and Attitudes* (Brown and Holtzman, 1969). Although these patients had all successfully completed some college level work, 95 percent of the subtest scores for the group fell below the 25th percentile for college freshmen. This points to a severe disturbance of habit patterns.

SUGGESTIONS FOR TREATMENT

It is apparent from the above formulation that the primary occupational dysfunction of the borderline patient occurs at the level of exploratory behavior, or play, and becomes evident in the inability to perform autonomous adult roles. The vicious cycle which has arrested the system must be modified. How can this be done in the context of adult activity and pre-vocational groups? How can patients acquire the playfulness they need to work?

First, a setting which makes clear, consistent functional demands within a specific time frame is necessary to allow for the development of a benign cycle of work behaviors. This provides both the safe environment necessary for the emergence of spontaneous work and play, and a predictable setting to practice adult roles. Most prevocational settings provide this adequately.

Second, while the functional demands are clearly delineated, the context for fulfilling these demands needs to be one of exploration, acceptance, and curiosity about the doing process. The program is an arena for the patients to experience themselves in action. It provides an opportunity for them to mobilize and appreciate their genuinely creative and productive capacities, as well as an opportunity to become aware of unproductive patterns, and explore strategies for change. Initiative is encouraged and nurtured. The most important factor in creating such an environment is the role of the occupational therapist. She is neither a therapist nor a boss. She holds functional expectations, but does not measure success solely on the basis of achievement of these expectations. Rather she holds a space and provides encouragement for the patient to struggle with meeting and failing to meet expectations. She notices and appreciates genuineness. The health apprentice role proposed by Burke, Miyake, Kielhofner, and Barris, (1983), which stresses patients' learning new skills, and reorganizing life tasks around exploration of alternatives, decision making, and problem solving, comes closest to the role suggested here. The most important thing the occupational therapist can do for the borderline patient is model, appreciate and mirror a lively process of active self-exploration and experimentation with new strategies, while simultaneously ensuring the safety of the environment.

Example one: Nancy was a rigid, perfectionistic borderline adolescent. She feared many activities. When she attempted tasks or schoolwork, she would quit in a rage at the first signs of difficulty. Avoidant or self destructive behavior often followed. With the occupational therapist's assistance Nancy developed some challenging enamelling tasks. The occupational therapist made it clear that Nancy's effort to generate multiple strategies for dealing with problems which might arise was more important than successfully completing the task. She was readily available to consult with Nancy, and vetoed several ideas which could have been dangerous or frustrating. The game was, "How many things can go wrong, and how many ways can I find of fixing them?" Winning was taking risks and trying original ideas while tolerating uncertainty and failure. Slowly Nancy began to build an exploratory base for more flexible task behavior.

Example two: Donna expressed a need to improve her typing speed and initiative in order to return to work. She often complained of feeling dead at her clerical jobs. At the same time she had vibrant, unrealized fantasies of being an actress or artist. The occupational therapist encouraged her to design a project, involving typing, which really appealed to her. Donna chose to type out and illustrate a recurrent fantasy as a children's story. Donna showed more initiative and extended activity engagement in implementing this task than had been evident in several years of occupational therapy treatment. The uniqueness of her delicate watercolors was noted appreciatively by both patients and staff. She expressed pleasure and pride in her work and produced a higher caliber end product. She independently made plans for additional books.

The more borderline patients come directly into contact with exploratory activity and receive the resultant intrinsic and extrinsic gratification, the more volitional system modification will occur and more stable habit patterns evolve.

The St. Luke's Day Treatment Program's activity/pre-vocational component was designed to maximize exploratory opportunities. There are three "doing" groups: a project group, a dance movement group, and a student group. Each has clear functional expectations, while placing a strong emphasis on the members' ability to notice and become curious about their process. For example, in the student group, there are grades, assignments and tests to simulate a college classroom environment. However, members write down their impressions of the process after each assignment and there are weekly writing and thinking exercises which are purely exploratory. The groups are offered in three month semesters to enable patients to change groups as their needs or goals change. Group choice is made by consensus of patient and counselor. At the end of each semester all day program members and staff meet as a group to evaluate the groups which have ended and share hopes and goals for the new groups.

There are two pre-vocational groups which occur in a graded sequence. The work image group entails completely exploratory activities and assignments dealing with work history, fantasies, choices, and skills. Techniques used in the group include formal and informal assessments, process writing, and activities. Members enter the practical issues group when they are ready for some work involvement outside the program. It focuses on acquiring the skills necessary to perform the worker role; i.e., interviewing, resumé writing, handling authority and peer work relationships. Extensive use is made of volunteer jobs, which are done outside of program hours. These jobs often provide the widest range of exploration and allow patients to practice different vocational plans in a realistic way. As members begin to have real work experiences, continued open-ended exploration of work issues occurs in the group.

Through exploration and pleasurable engagement with activity, patients gradually become less impulsive and more resilient. Rather than fleeing when faced with a difficult situation, a patient might notice himself wanting to leave, take a break to write down reactions, return to work, and discuss his experiences at the end of the group. Slowly, new values develop and goals become tempered by reality.

Case Study

Anita is a 30-year-old religious, Catholic woman. She is the youngest of three children. Both parents are alcoholic and the history reveals an extremely erratic homelife. She and her siblings were periodically abused.

Her vocational background is in musical performance. She has not performed professionally, but has received a BA in performance and pursued graduate course work in that area. She also has good clerical skills. After a brief, unhappy marriage, she separated from her husband, became unable to perform due to severe anxiety, and took a leave of absence from school. During this time she was hospitalized briefly on two occasions. After the second hospitalization, she entered the day program. Her vocational goal at that time was to return to school.

Anita was assigned to the newspaper project group and to the prevocational image group. Her initial externally directed use of activity was apparent in the newspaper group, where following the rules, pleasing the leader, and becoming the best member were her major considerations. Gradually, with encouragement, she was able to derive satisfaction from writing about subjects which interested her. In the work image group she recognized how she used her music to impress others, particularly a "father figure" teacher. She was encouraged to take an improvisation class and followed up on this. She decided to explore career options outside of music, such as nursing. When Anita applied for volunteer jobs as nurse's aide she learned quickly that this was not a genuine interest but a helping fantasy. Further exploration of helping roles was then carried out through Anita's election as community chairperson. In this role she mobilized many organizational strengths and was able to feel genuine pleasure in her productivity and capacity to help others.

At this point Anita had incorporated some new elements into her system of occupational behavior. She had a taste of the potential satisfaction of productivity, and she had explored different career options which allowed her to feel more solid in her choice of music. However, her intense need to please others and her extrinsic motivation were still apparent. She felt empty and terrified at giving up the grandiose musician self to which she had clung.

Three selections from Anita's process writing at this time reveal her painful confrontation of her musician fantasy, and the resultant chaos as her old volitional system structure crumbled. "I wanted to get a Doctorate in performing. I am disappointed in my nervous condition which will prevent me from doing this. I can't go back to the pressures which made me sick, so what in the hell am I to do now? I'm terrified of this improvisation class. I am out of shape pianistically, and my hands are stiff with medication."

"Most of the time I was alone, all-alone alone. In the house and in the park, I was alone. I feel that aloneness now, that uncertainty— anything could happen. Life is unpredictable. I never knew what to expect in my house when I came through the door . . . "

"I am always trying to get their love and attention. I only succeed when I achieve something. Then they think I'm great. I, in and of myself, am valueless. I am only in life to entertain and give."

Anita was in a difficult intermediate stage. She was ready to abandon old values but had not yet recognized or claimed new ones. At this point, the new school semester started and she chose to return to full time work and school. As she had feared, the pressure was too great. Her symptoms worsened, requiring a brief re-hospitalization. She lost her job, but was able to continue her course work and returned to the day program.

Anita continued the painful process reflected in her writing. There was, however, a new flexibility and openness to alternatives. She began to talk in great detail, and with conviction, of wanting to take care of herself. She found herself wanting to be able to afford nice clothing and vacations. This change of focus signaled the completion of a genuine volitional system alteration. Her sense of herself and her abilities was more realistic and integrated. Additionally, self-care and leisure interests were blossoming. Within several months, Anita left the day program for full time work with a religious organization she valued. Her immediate desire was to support herself, with a long term goal of returning to a musical career.

Eight months after treatment Anita was still at her job. She took pride in her excellent ratings. She had recently received one promotion, and was going to be trained in word processing. She hoped shortly to be making enough money to rent a piano for practicing and teaching.

SUMMARY

A formulation of borderline occupational functioning was developed using the model of human occupation as a theoretical framework. A treatment approach derived from this formulation is delineated. The need for a setting which makes clear, consistent functional demands is noted. The role of the occupational therapist in creating a context of curious exploration as functional demands are addressed, is stressed. One specific treatment program is described and the therapeutic change process is illustrated through clinical case examples.

The empirical validity of this theoretical formulation needs to be investigated through studies of the play and habit histories of borderline patients. Also, the effectiveness of the treatment approach needs be evaluated through follow-up studies of work success.

REFERENCE NOTES

1. Kielhofner, G., Personal Communication, April 7, 1983.
2. Salz, C. & White, S. *The St. Luke's Acute Day Treatment Program Pre-Vocational Questionnaire.* Unpublished evaluation form, 1983.

REFERENCES

Burke, J.P., Miyake, S., Kielkofner, G., & Barris, R. The demystification of health care and demise of the sick role: implications for occupational therapy. In G. Kielhofner (Ed.), *Health through Occupation: Theory and Practice in Occupational Therapy.* Philadelphia: F.A. Davis, 1983.

Brown, W. & Holtzman, W.H. *Survey of Study Habits and Attitudes* (Test Materials). New York: The Psychological Corporation, 1964.

Fast, Irene. Aspects of work style and work difficulty in borderline personalities. *International Journal of Psychoanalysis*, 1975, *56*, 397-403.

Kernberg, O. *Borderline Conditions and Pathological Narcissism*. New York: Jason Aronson, Inc., 1975.

Kielhofner, G. A model of human occupation, part two. Ontogenesis from the perspective of temporal adaptation. *The American Journal of Occupational Therapy*, 1980, *34*, 657-663.

Kielhofner, G. & Burke, J.P. A model of human occupation, part 1. Structure and content, *The American Journal of Occupational Therapy*, 1980, *34*, 572-581.

Mahler, M.S., Pine, F., & Bergman, A. *The Psychological Birth of the Human Infant*. New York: Basic Books, 1975.

Rinsley, D.B. An object-relations view of borderline personality. In P. Hartocollis (Ed.), *Borderline Personality Disorders: The Concept, The Syndrome, The Patient*. New York: International Universities Press, Inc., 1977.

Sass, L. The borderline personality. *The New York Times Magazine*, August 22, 1982, pp. 15-18; 66-67.

Stern, D. The first relationship: infant and mother. In Bruner, J., Cole, M., & Lloyd, B. (Eds.) *The Developing Child*. Cambridge: Harvard University Press, 1977.

Sutherland, J.D. The British object-relations theorists: Balint, Winnicott, Fairbairn, Guntrip, *Journal of the American Psychoanalytic Association*, 1980, *28*, 829-860.

Winnicott, D. W. Ego distortion in terms of true and false self (1960). In D.W. Winnicott (collected papers), *the Maturational Processes and the Facilitating Environment*. New York: International Universities Press, 1965.

Winnicott, D.W. The theory of the parent infant relationship (1960). In D.W. Winnicott (collected papers), *the Maturational Processes and the Facilitating Environment*. New York: International Universities Press, 1965.

Winnicott, D.W. *Playing and Reality*. New York: Basic Books, 1975.

Inpatient Management
of the Borderline Patient

Carol A. Kaplan, MS, RNCS

ABSTRACT. Patients with a borderline personality organization evoke unique problems and treatment dilemmas among members of an inpatient treatment team. The first section of this article addresses the many problems and complexities involved in the management of borderline patients in an intensive inpatient psychiatric setting. The second section describes guidelines, approaches, and therapeutic interventions aimed at reducing destructive influences and maximizing treatment outcome.

PROBLEMS IN MANAGING THE BORDERLINE PATIENT

Patients with a borderline personality organization have unique character problems that make treatment extremely difficult. A tumultuous course of hospitalization is characterized frequently by repeated self-destructive and other acting-out behavior, a complex splitting process between the patient and the hospital social structure, and growing tension and conflict among staff. Some cases develop into an escalating, contagiously destructive spiral which eventually results in the discharge or transfer of the borderline patient in intense turmoil; leaving behind a severely fragmented treatment team struggling to resolve its differences.

What is it about the borderline patient that makes inpatient management so complex, problematic, and entangled with provocative treatment dilemmas? Patients with a borderline personality organization are often negativistic, demanding, self-destructive, and prone to a multitude of acting-out behaviors within a therapeutic milieu. Furthermore, these patients manifest: little capacity for anxiety, poor frustration tolerance, an inability to tolerate delay, and poor impulse control. They frequently have an insatiable need for special

---

Carol A. Kaplan is Assistant Director in the Nursing Department at The Sheppard and Enoch Pratt Hospital in Towson, Maryland.

attention, and they enter the psychiatric unit communicating a sense of entitlement which evokes angry reactions from patients and staff. They present an exquisite sensitivity to rejection and criticism, as well as a suspicion and mistrust which often barely falls short of a bona fide paranoia. Borderline patients also frequently express the need to control and to be controlled and the need to exploit and to be exploited.[1,2]

The aforementioned behaviors present a challenging clinical picture, but such a cluster does not provide a complete explanation of what is so uniquely complex about treating the borderline patient. The significant dynamic features which distinguish the problems in management of the borderline patient involve the defense mechanisms of splitting and projective identification. Treatment teams comprised of highly skilled, clinically sophisticated staff members can be torn asunder by this defensive structure; hence providing a reenactment of the inconsistent, frustrating, and, at times, rejecting environment of the patient's earlier years.[3]

Projective identification is a process in which the patient projects various parts of himself onto various staff members. These staff members are often appealed to at a level outside of their awareness, and they may therefore act, or feel like acting, like the projected parts. For example, a patient projects onto a staff member cruel, punishing parts of himself. The projection reverberates with something in the staff member which had been submerged, and the staff member will tend to react to the patient in a cruel, sadistic, and punishing manner. Likewise, staff who have received idealized projected parts of the patient will tend to respond in an overly involved, protective, indulgent manner.[4] An example of projective identification can be demonstrated by an interaction the author recently had with a nurse. Ms. T was describing her relationship with a borderline patient who had been on the unit for approximately three weeks. She explained that the patient had become negativistic and increasingly demanding, stating that her demands had no bounds. She then said that for the past week, the patient had been constantly referring to Ms. T as "Nurse Ratchett," and if that was not difficult enough, the patient was also regaling new patients on the unit about what a tyrant Ms. T was. Further inquiring made it clear that soon after the patient had cast Ms. T into "Nurse Ratchett's" role, Ms. T started to react to the patient in a far more rigid manner than is typical for her, and indeed, the bulk of her interactions with the patient were now focused on policy adherence and strict limit setting. Although outside of her awareness, Ms. T was on her way to repeating a script straight out of the movie, "One Flew Over the Cuckoo's Nest."

Describing the process of splitting in an inpatient setting, both positive and negative aspects of the patient's feelings are projected onto different staff members, some of whom are seen as good and helpful, and others as bad and destructive. Frequently, the borderline patient judges staff members as being all good or all bad following a very brief acquaintance.[5] The fluidity of role casting is also noteworthy, and it is not unusual for the long sought after "knight in shining armor" to be cast into the role of a cruel, horrible person an hour later. The mechanisms of splitting and projective identification help explain why different staff members see the same patient in very different ways.

Soon after the patient is admitted to the hospital, staff splitting is likely to begin if staff members become the recipients of the patient's externalized conflict.[6] The projection of the positive and negative feelings onto the environment divides the staff into two groups when this externalization takes place. An example of this process:

> Oh, Mr. R is an inappropriate admission. Really, I don't know what he's doing in a place like this. I hear that he never established any kind of a therapeutic alliance during his last, rather lengthy, hospitalization, and in fact, he was finally asked to leave because of heavy drug dealing. It doesn't seem to me as if anything has changed. He's already hostile, manipulative, and demanding, and he doesn't seem the least bit motivated to get into treatment.

A different staff member's response when asked about the same patient:

> Well, I had a long talk with Mr. R today, and he seems quite depressed. Judging from his previous records, it sounds as if he's in a much different place this time. He was telling me about all of his family problems, and it sounds as though his parents have flat out rejected him.

Herein lies the beginning of a destructive splitting process which, in the case of Mr. R, would soon become an extremely difficult treatment situation. T.F. Main refers to this good and bad split as the formation of the "In group and the Out group."[7] Staff members in the In group engage upon a relationship with the patient which becomes closer than usual, and they have frequent discussions with the therapist outside of the usual team meetings and case conferences which concern the patient. These staff members are regarded by the patient and themselves as having a special understanding of the patient's difficulties. Characteristic perpetuating features of this group are: the sentimental appeal from the patient ("I need you, you are my lifeline, you make me feel complete"),[8] and in turn, the compelling arousal of omnipotence in the staff member. Special privileges and excessive time and attention are required of this individual by the patient and by the In group around him. These staff members become much more permissive and tolerant of the patient's special demands than is typical for them, and their approach to the patient starts to become less dictated by their clinical judgments grounded in theory and more by the patient's behavior. While these In-group interactional processes are gaining momentum and intensity, staff in the Out group are either openly disagreeing with the In group—or they're talking among themselves with increasing criticism and blame of the In group's handling of the situation. The Out group accuses the In group of being collusive, unrealistic, overindulgent, and ineffectual at limit-setting, whereas the In group speaks of the Out group as being rigid, punitive, suppressive, and insensitive to the patient's psychic pain.[9] It is not unusual for every treatment team member as well as some people outside of the treatment team to become aligned with a warring camp, each convinced that the other is totally mistaken concerning how the patient should be treated.[10] In the meantime, the patient is likely to become increasingly disturbed, and this is frequently evidenced by acting-out and self-destructive behavior. The other patients on the unit are also not impervious to the destructive influences of this growing dissension. The effects of this process among the patient group can be manifested in several ways: increased acting out, withdrawal, fragmentation of the patient group which often parallels staff In-and-Out groups, and group scapegoating of the special patient. Additionally, there may be expressed veneration towards the patient with encouragement of and participation in his destructive behavior on the unit. Left unchecked, this devastating process eventually becomes unbearable for everyone involved. It is at this juncture that most often, the borderline patient is transferred to another facility, and this action is usually enough to rapidly restore some semblance of equilibrium to the milieu. Everyone has paid a price however, and unless much time and effort goes into attempting to understand the various components of this escalating spiral, it is reasonable to predict that the stage has been set for a repeat performance with a slightly modified cast.

There is much controversy in the literature surrounding the question of who triggers off whom in the splitting process. That is, does the borderline patient, given his proclivity to splitting, fall victim to preexisting staff conflict, or can the patient indeed be the lone provocateur of such upheaval in a system that does not already have its roots embedded in unresolved intra- and interstaff conflicts? Is the patient the catalyst or the powerful initiator? This question can easily lead to the pitfall of finger pointing and blame seeking which serves no useful purpose. Nonetheless, it deserves some consideration. It is the author's opinion that it can go both ways. That is, a severely borderline patient can pave the way to serious splitting in a treatment team that is quite cohesive, and a team that functions maturely in the area of conflict resolution. This view is not supported by Stanton and Schwartz, who place primary emphasis on the hospital's contribution to the problem.[11] The author also believes however that at times, the patient mobilizes splits which had been submerged in and among staff members. The patient is very sensitive to already existing conflict, and he knows how to manipulate. Common underlying conflicts which already exist in the system, and usually get mobilized by the system are:

1. Covert conflict between different departments within the hospital (e.g., medical and nursing).
2. Intradepartmental conflict at various hierarchical levels (e.g., medical supervisors and residents).
3. A conflict of ideologies (e.g., a family therapy orientation versus an individual, analytical approach to treatment).
4. Feelings of resentment and competition between the formal and informal decision-making structures within the hospital.
5. Latent conflict among staff on the unit (e.g., the novice staff member who resents the alleged rigidity of the head nurse and is therefore particularly vulnerable to forming a splitting alliance with the patient.)[12]

Book, Sadavoy, and Silver describe five common countertransference responses that the borderline patient tends to evoke in staff:[13]

1. *The patient "Bad" vs. the patient "Troubled."* That is, there is frequently the temptation to assess the patient as being manipulative and uncooperative rather than troubled, frightened, and possibly desperate. The patient who, upon admission, covers over his abandonment depression with a veneer of arrogance is sometimes labeled a manipulative psychopath who does not belong in the hospital.

2. *The staff person who feels he can do no wrong.* This stance occurs as a result of projective identification in which the borderline patient projects his all-good objects onto a staff member, hence creating an idealization of that staff person. The staff member receives gratification from this position, and may unknowingly maintain the idealization. This is often manifested by colluding with unrealistic demands made by the patient.

3. *Intrastaff fragmentation and intrapatient conflicts.* Again, this refers to the phenomena of staff acting out the patient's intrapsychic conflicts through the mechanism of projective identification and splitting.

4. *Feelings of hopelessness in patients and staff.* Feelings of hopelessness are often communicated by the borderline patient as he begins to experience abandonment depression. Although this is not unique to the borderline patient, intense feelings of hopelessness may resonate in staff, and they may react by withdrawing from the patient at such times.

5. *Therapeutic limit setting vs. sadistic control.* Limit setting may trigger conflicts relating to one's own aggression, and in an attempt to deal with these conflicts, staff may become either uncaringly lax or controllingly punitive around the issue of limit setting. Such extreme staff postures often become complicating features of inpatient treatment of the borderline individual. A lax approach to limit setting does not provide the patient with needed external controls, and it serves as an open invitation to regression. For example, Mr. R starts flaunting minor infractions, and staff members, while exasperated with his behavior, fail to take a firm stand and set limits consistently. Perhaps they don't want to stir him up ("after all, it's so minor"), or maybe they're beginning to question themselves over what undoubtedly will be the patient's response (i.e., "you're all just picking on me again"), or possibly this represents a covert

wish on the part of staff to get rid of the patient. In any case, an unspoken ground rule is established between staff and patient whereby only more serious actions will result in direct interventions. Of course, Mr. R responds to this treatment posture by escalating his acting-out behavior, and before long, he's engaged in far more serious, destructive behavior. This scenario oftentimes creates a situation of discharge or a crisis around limit setting with possible punishment for the patient.

A controlling approach to limit setting, on the other hand, which is guided by rigid, absolute restrictions, tends to create incessant power struggles between the staff and patient. This can become the total focus of treatment, whereby the patient fails to address the problems that brought him into the hospital. The borderline patient will not experience his anxieties, inner turmoil, and depression as long as all of his energies are invested in maintaining an adversarial relationship with the staff.[14]

It has often been said that one of the major weaknesses of the borderline individual lies in his proneness to regression, while one of the strengths is his ability to reverse the process. The regressive pull is frequently intensified in an inpatient setting, and this rather striking clinical feature is another significant complexity of nursing management of the borderline patient. Arnold Modell discusses the patient's reaction to hospitalization in terms of the patient's relationship with his therapist: "The therapist is perceived invariably as one endowed with magical, omnipotent qualities, who will, merely by his contact with a patient, affect a cure without the necessity of the patient to be active or responsible."[15] In terms of Modell's description, hospitalization provides a multitude of such potential therapists. That is, everyone involved in the patient's treatment can be perceived by the patient as a potential source of magical relief, and also a potential trigger for the disappointment that inevitably follows when the magical wish is not fulfilled. Hence, the very structure of an intensive treatment setting, which demands active engagement of staff and patients, contains the elements for destructive regression.

The borderline patient's typical response to hospitalization is an initial rapid infantile regression and dependence on the staff which is then followed by destructive acting out when the wish for immediate relief does not occur.[16] This is a somewhat accentuated repetition of the patient's longstanding pattern in interpersonal relationships, that is, relationships which fluctuate according to an uncommunicated need state, and which end in disillusionment when the need is not met. Severe regression soon after hospitalization is characterized by: anger and rage through mutism, self-inflicted lacerations, verbal and physical abuse of staff, window breaking, overt sexual acting out, drug taking, destruction of property, acquisition of drugs for other patients, encouragement of destructive behavior by other, more regressed patients, and other various types of behaviors in which to a greater or lesser degree threaten the structure and boundaries which have been designed to provide a safety zone for patients and staff.[17] Self-destructive behavior, in particular, often sets up an escalating spiral between the staff and patient which ultimately serves to reinforce the borderline personality organization. This process can be conceptualized in the following way: The patient's frustrated wish for the omnipotent, magical helper contributes to self-destructive behavior. Hospital staff members often respond to such behavior by increasing hospital care through ward restrictions and constant observation. This response tends to reinforce the patient's wish for total care, and he will tend to do whatever is necessary to maintain this care, hence setting up a model in which further acting-out behavior and regression is perpetuated. As this pattern continues, staff tend to become angry and frustrated at the patient. The attitude of some staff members may swing from that of support and protective concern to anger which is expressed through withdrawal or retaliation. Simultaneously, the patient is perjoratively labeled a manipulator or an attention seeker. This polarized reactivity on the part of staff closely duplicates the twin themes of the parental-child interaction, which are characterized by clinging closeness and rejecting withdrawal. Unless this self-perpetuating cycle is interrupted, it is likely that the borderline patient will find himself becoming more chaotic and more self-destructive during intensive treatment than he had been prior to hospitalization.[18]

TREATMENT GUIDELINES, APPROACHES, AND INTERVENTIONS

The planning and implementation of various approaches aimed at minimizing the potential for destructive interplay between the patient's personality structure and the hospital social structure is a vitally important aspect of the treatment regime. Therapeutic change in the borderline patient occurs only when he no longer receives the same old signals from the same old objects. Herein lies the challenge for staff to offer the patient a new kind of experience rather than reconfirming the projections he is so expert in eliciting from people. What measures need to be taken in order to provide the patient with such a corrective experience?

The first crucial step is staff education. Staff members need to have a working understanding of the typical behavior profile of the borderline individual, key psychodynamic concepts, potential pitfalls of hospital treatment, and various strategies for avoiding these pitfalls. The staff member who does not understand splitting, for example, and the defensive function it serves for the patient, is far more likely to engage in a destructive dyad with the patient. Ideally, this education should occur when the treatment team is not already engaged in an emotionally laden entanglement with the borderline patient. However, teaching can certainly be effective when staff are in the midst of a splitting situation, and the experience itself can be used as an effective tool in facilitating an understanding of the various processes involved.[19,20]

A hospital structure which provides for free and open communication among team members is another important element which helps to promote a positive treatment experience for the borderline individual. How much support does the organization structure lend to ongoing, open, and honest interactional processes among staff? What attitudes surrounding conflict resolution filter down from higher levels within the hierarchy? Undoubtedly, these considerations have a potent and direct effect on the team's ability to unravel and sift through splitting entanglements when they do occur.[21]

Leadership and direction within the team is extremely important in helping to identify group issues and goals which will facilitate open communication among the team. Effective leadership is an essential component of a viable treatment plan for patients who use splitting.[22] These patients frequently were raised in families which had blurred generational boundaries; the parent-child axis at times being completely reversed.[23] Hence, leadership and group cohesion represent the integrated authority figure which the patient did not have.

The group leader needs to anticipate the splitting of the team as well as being attuned to the nuances and the more blatant countertransference responses of the team. It is most useful if he can serve as an arbitrator when splitting does occur, facilitating and supporting the group in their efforts toward resolution, thereby assisting the patient in reinternalizing the conflict. It is also incumbent upon the leader to be aware when outside consultation is indicated. An objective outsider's viewpoint is needed when the clinical leader loses perspective of the total group process and becomes involved in the splitting among staff.[24] The leader needs to watch for several danger signals which indicate emotional overinvolvement:[25]

1. Different staff members view a borderline patient in different ways, and the leader becomes convinced that Group A's perception is far more accurate than that of Group B.
2. The leader finds himself either assuming or supporting a treatment posture which is reflected by strict adherence to rigid rules or overly simplified treatment. Any thinking that starts out with "all you need to do is"—for example, "set firm and consistent limits," is usually a tell-tale sign.
3. The leader begins to share the burned-out, exhausted, hopeless feelings that staff are expressing about the management of a particular patient.
4. Staff starts talking about the therapist who has wrecked everything and left them to pick up the pieces, and the leader agrees.

Frequent staff meetings are crucial in developing trusting relationships among staff so that the patient's projections can be readily recognized for what they are. Staff members really need to know where each other stands on certain issues.[26] When staff member "A" knows and respects the clinical judgment of staff member "B," and the patient complains to "A" about the gross injustices of "B," "A" is likely to think that the patient is distorting, based on her genuine belief that "B" could not possibly have said or done what the patient alleges. "A" is then in a position in which she can help the patient negotiate appropriately with "B," and the patient can then be assisted in exploring the nature of her distortions.

In addition to staff meetings, it is important to have larger team conferences comprising all staff members who are directly involved with the patient's treatment. Current patient and patient-staff issues need to be open for scrutiny in these meetings. Furthermore, they should be designed in such a way as to encourage each participant to share his experiences with the patient and to voice his attitudes toward his colleagues, which may at times include feelings of mistrust and blame. When these group meetings succeed, they accomplish several purposes:

1. They serve to piece together a more coherent, whole picture of the patient. There are frequently many contradictory perceptions and observations from different team members about the patient. Close examination, however, often reveals the part truths of those various pieces, and this promotes a more accurate, comprehensive understanding of the borderline individual.
2. These meetings will also ameliorate each participant's sense of having private knowledge and a special understanding of the patient. It is not uncommon for staff members to discover that more than one of them had been entrusted with the same secret. Hence, individuals discover that they, in fact, had not been so singularly honored by the patient. This decreases the burden by those staff who had felt singled out, and it also reduces the temptation to assume an omnipotent rescuing role and the subsequent guilt and anger at being unable to fill it.
3. When In-and-Out groups have been formed, these meetings will help each group become more tolerant of the others' attitudes and approaches toward the patient. The In-group staff who have been cast in the all-good role tend to feel less honored and less indebted to repay the honor, while those seen as bad are usually better able to endure the patient's relentless bombardment.[27]

There will be times, despite productive meetings, when the fragmentation continues. This need not be viewed as a problem as long as there is an acknowledgement of In-and-Out groups, and staff realize that this represents the very dichotomy in the patient. What does constitute poor treatment however is when there is a lack of awareness that the factions exist, and competition between the two groups goes on covertly.

It is also essential that individual staff members be on guard for their own cues that they're losing perspective and that they seek objective consultation at such times. As Main so beautifully states, ''It has been well said that the trouble with self-analysis lies in the countertransference. The help of another in the review of one's unconscious processes is a much better safeguard.''[28] The borderline patient is provocative, manipulative, and he has an almost uncanny ability to hone in on and exaggerate one's personal idiosyncrasies. Unless the staff member can clearly understand just what the patient is doing and how it is affecting his own emotions, he will not be able to deal with the patient therapeutically.

Obvious as it may seem, the first step toward successful management of the borderline patient involves an accurate assessment that the patient does indeed have a borderline personality organization. Borderline patients are often initially diagnosed based on their rather glaring presenting symptoms.[29] Examples of this would include patients who are diagnosed as having anorexia nervosa, obsessive-compulsive personality, sociopathic personality, hysterical personality, or anxiety neuroses. An early, accurate diagnosis is essential to the patient and the staff who will be working with him. Treatment based upon a misdiagnosis often leads to chronic regressive responses in the patient. This is demonstrated by the following vignette:

> Ms. W was a 31-year-old, single female admitted to the hospital with a diagnosis of obsessive-compulsive personality. The presenting symptomatology which was most striking was her excessive ritualistic behavior around activities involving self-hygiene and the avoidance of contamination by others. Her hands were scrubbed raw, and if permitted, Ms. W would devote most of her day to her hand-washing rituals. Soon after admission, Ms. W became extremely angry, demanding, and manipulative. She rapidly acquired the status of special patient on the unit. More and more time and attention was being devoted to her, and she soon became the focus of discussion in many staff meetings, service conferences and community meetings. Ms. W's behavior gave rise to staff splitting with the formation of classical in groups and out groups within the treatment team. Some staff members treated her in an overly protective manner, which seemed quite infantilizing. They frequently responded to her demandingness by immediately complying. Other staff members adamantly expressed the need for firm limit setting, and while this was certainly indicated, their ideas about this seemed to be overly rigid and suppressive. It was not long before Ms. W's internal conflicts were being heatedly acted out among an increasingly conflicted, fragmented staff group. An objective consultant was called in to review the case, and it was he who changed the patient's

diagnosis to that of borderline personality organization. This had an almost immediate remedying effect among the treatment team, as they were now better able to take a more objective view of the splitting which had occurred, and they could understand this process in the context of the patient's pathology. Group meetings were held which included everyone involved in Ms. W's treatment. Effective limits were established and consistently enforced, the patient's ritualistic behavior was defocused as much as possible, and the patient no longer succeeded in playing one staff member off against another. The patient responded well to the modified approach, and core borderline dilemmas soon began to emerge as her abandonment depression surfaced. Ms. W was later discharged in a much improved condition.

When the borderline individual is admitted to the hospital, the initial treatment goal is often that of protecting and stabilizing the patient. An evaluation that carefully assesses the patient's need for protection must be done immediately.[30] Sometimes, the borderline individual will verbally express suicidal ideation or self-destructive thoughts. However, quite often these patients have a capacity to present a "false self" picture that minimizes their current desperation and risk of self-harm. Affect may convey more than words when an inquiry is made regarding the patient's suicidal potential. It's most important to be attuned to any inappropriate affect with perceptive acuity. This initial assessment should also include a determination of previous destructive behaviors; the patient's view of precipitating events leading to hospitalization; and a history of recent losses, either fantasized or real. An accurate assessment of the patient's needs at the beginning of hospitalization, and an implementation of necessary protective and supportive measures by staff, (e.g., locked ward, special observations if necessary) often quickly result in a dramatic reduction of the patient's sense of panic.[31]

Once the basic protective needs of the patient are met, a more comprehensive evaluation of the patient can occur. This is necessary in order to develop an individualized treatment plan based on a more thorough understanding of the psychological profile the patient has carried with him to the hospital. Staff members need to learn more about the patient's previous dysfunctional patterns of behavior, thus enabling them to help the patient connect those to the here and now when the behaviors are reenacted in the milieu. Likewise, it is equally important to find out about the patient's more functional behavioral patterns, and more adaptive coping mechanisms in order to appeal to his inner strengths. This evaluation involves close collaboration with the entire treatment team. Holistic treatment cannot occur if, for example, nursing staff members and the family therapist are not working together very closely. A recent research study indicates that a consistent pattern of neglect and a reliance on denial characterize the familial situation of borderline offspring.[32] The patient's symptomatology often serves a valuable function in maintaining the family equilibrium, and the family's regressive pull is often phenomenal. When the family is made an integral part of the patient's treatment, the benefits of hospitalization are far less likely to be undermined by threatened family members. Additionally, the borderline patient tends to distort intrafamilial relationships, and this distortion often leads to splitting. A collaborative involvement with the family and the family therapist helps to clarify such perceptual distortions and minimize splitting tendencies.

Included in the patient assessment, staff members need to evaluate the patient's regressive potential, and a therapeutic approach that addresses itself to this potential must then be formulated. An intensive treatment setting seems to promote regression and self-destructive acting out unless behavioral limits are defined clearly and early in the hospitalization. All authors advocate limit setting within a supportive framework as a means of minimizing regressive behavior. Depending upon the hospital's philosophy of treatment, it is sometimes useful to negotiate a preadmission contract with the patient, wherein the patient knows what is expected of him and what he can expect of others. The limits, in effect, become a statement of what the hospital has to offer.[33]

The manner in which staff approach limit setting can make the difference between a productive hospital experience and one that is either nonproductive or counterproductive. Angry, punitive limit setting merely confirms the patient's expectations. Suppressive and rigid limits create obstacles to self-exploration and therapeutic change. This approach also confirms the patient's notion that he has little or no control over his life situation. It is essential that staff not view the limits and expectations as their controls over the patient. For example, a borderline patient engages in physically aggressive acting-out behavior: One way of dealing with this might be to emphasize the need for medications and to tighten up ward restrictions. The team might also issue an ultimatum, such as, "One more similar episode, and we're going to have to transfer you to another hospital.''

Another way of approaching the situation could be: ''I can't understand why you're putting the treatment team in the position of having to reassess continuation of your stay in this hospital. Has there been some change in your feelings about helping yourself?''[34]

Clearly, the difference in the latter approach is that it reinforces the idea that the patient has a definite role in his life situation, and the control and the decisions reside with him. It also communicates to the patient an attitude of respect which could be a boost to his self-esteem. The more the staff are able to align themselves with the nonregressed aspects of the patient's ego, the better are the chances for improved functioning.

The milieu can be very effective in helping the patient counteract the regressive pull, as well as providing the patient with an experience in which he can gain insight into his behavior. Aside from what the staff tells him, the borderline patient will rapidly get a sense from other patients on the unit of the level of acting out which will be tolerated. The patient will respond positively to a well-functioning milieu in which mature, responsible behavior is the expectation. The therapeutic community must adopt a position towards the acting out of the borderline individual, and a process needs to be facilitated whereby both staff and patients are involved in limit setting. In order for this to occur, of course, staff members need to help the other patients understand that firm limit setting is indeed in the best interest of the patient.[35] Milieu work with the borderline individual is most effective if it focuses upon the reality of expectations, the process of decision-making, and interactional behaviors and dynamics in the here and now.

It is the author's opinion that medications should be used most sparingly in spite of frequent temptations to do otherwise. These patients typically will do almost anything to avoid experiencing their psychic pain. This pattern gets reinforced if, when the patient experiences abandonment depression, he is given a pill to alleviate the pain. The patient needs to know that the feelings are not going to destroy him and also that people will respond to his needs and lend emotional support when he needs it. Also, borderline individuals oftentimes have a history of drug abuse, and treating drug abusers with medications can be a sticky business. Lastly, the use of medications serves to further reinforce the message that the patient is sick, not in control, and not responsible for his own behavior. The author finds it questionable to use psychotropic medications in treating borderline patients unless the individual's anxiety is so monumental that he cannot progress without it, or if the patient is in a transient psychosis with disorganized thinking.

The process of termination is a vitally important phase of treatment for the borderline individual. The patient should have ample time to work this through. The patient should be an active participant in team discussions concerning discharge planning, and everyone involved should agree upon the actual date of discharge. The patient may experience regressive feelings as termination approaches, and it is frequently a mistake to react to this by deciding that the patient is really not ready to leave the hospital.[36,37] This action not only reinforces destructive parent-child interactions from the patient's earlier years, but it often sets the stage for the individual to become a revolving door patient for years to come. Hence, when the patient bellows a last minute plea to stay a little longer, it is crucial that this plea not be granted and that staff takes a firm stand on what the patient can do for himself. If the patient, in spite of all efforts, is too regressed to leave on the specified date, transfer to a larger custodial facility should be seriously considered.

There are several very specific techniques in treating borderline patients which are enumerated as follows:

1. Help the patient connect his thoughts and feelings to actions.
2. Clarify perceptual distortions with the patient at the time they occur.
3. Do not be manipulated into believing in the patient's helplessness.
4. Always help the patient keep in mind the immediate goals of the hospitalization based on what it was that brought him to the hospital.
5. Realize the necessity of dealing with the here and now rather than the patient's early childhood.
6. Resist the temptation to give in to the patient in order to forestall explosions.
7. Help the patient increase his frustration tolerance and impulse control.
8. Point out to the patient that he is pushing you by his ever increasing demands. His unrealistic feelings of entitlement must be exposed, and his manipulations must be consistently confronted.

9. Clarify the ward's limits, guidelines, and expectations when the patient is admitted.
10. Support and encourage steps toward individuation. Encourage the patient to make his own choices and decisions. Also encourage him to pursue his own interests. Do not always push the patient to do more, because some skepticism as to his abilities can motivate him in a positive direction.
11. Provide as constant an experience as possible.
12. Help the patient in the process of reinternalizing his conflicts. When he complains to one person about another, redirect him to the source. Also interpret the patient's projections: e.g., "Could it be that it's difficult for you to have these angry suspicious feelings, and you put these feelings onto me as a way of protecting yourself?"
13. Encourage verbalization as an alternative to acting out.
14. Confrontations should be firm and consistent without being angry.
15. Do not take an overly directive approach to meet the patient's dependency needs.
16. Consistently confront bizarre behavior.
17. Always confront the patient who consciously lies.
18. Provide external structure to decrease acting out.
19. Supervise family visits in order to gain a better understanding of their mutually pathogenic communications.
20. Always be aware of and responsive to the patient's strengths and self-esteem issues.
21. The appropriate use of humor can be useful in helping the patient maintain some distance from his feeling state.
22. Respond to the patient's urgent demands by asking the question of what makes it urgent. If the staff member acknowledges that he is bewildered and not clear why he should do what the patient is asking, the burden of thought and decision-making is placed back onto the patient.

In conclusion, the author is not suggesting that by minimizing staff splitting and projective identification, borderline patients will be assured of having a positive treatment outcome. Oftentimes, there is little or no progress in spite of excellent treatment efforts. What the author is suggesting however is that is is essential to do everything possible to provide the patient with the therapeutic experience of a corrective environment in which harmful complications of hospitalization are minimized and through which change can occur.

REFERENCES

1. Zetzel, E. A Developmental Approach to the Borderline Patient. *American Journal of Psychiatry,* 1971, 127:867-871.
2. Shapiro, E. R. The Psychodynamics and Developmental Psychology of the Borderline Patient: A Review of the Literature. *American Journal of Psychiatry,* 1978, 135:1305-1315.
3. Grunebaum, H., and Klerman, G. Wrist Slashing. *American Journal of Psychiatry,* 1967, 124:113-120.
4. Adler, G. Hospital Treatment of Borderline Patients. *American Journal of Psychiatry,* 1973, 130:32-35.
5. Kernberg, O. The Treatment of Patients with Borderline Personality Organization. *International Journal of Psycho-Analysis,* 1968, 59:600-619.
6. Carsar, D. The Defense Mechanism of Splitting: Developmental Origins, Effects on Staff, Recommendations for Nursing Care. *Journal of Psychiatric Nursing and Mental Health Services,* 1979, 17:21-28.
7. Main, T. F. The Ailment. *British Journal of Medical Psychology,* 1957, 30:129-145.
8. Burnham, D. D. The Special-Problem Patient: Victim or Agent of Splitting? *Psychiatry,* 1966, 29:105-122.
9. Main, T. F., 1957.
10. Burnham, D. L., 1966.
11. Stanton, A. and Schwartz, M. *The Mental Hospital,* New York: Basic Books, Inc., 1954.
12. Burnham, D. L., 1966.
13. Book, H., Sadavoy, J., and Silver, D. Staff Countertransference to Borderline Patients on an Inpatient Unit. *American Journal of Psychotherapy,* 1978, 32:521-531.
14. Adler, G., 1973.
15. Wishnie, H. A. Inpatient Therapy with Borderline Patients. In *Borderline States in Psychiatry,* Mack, J. E. (Ed.) New York: Grune and Stratton, 1975, 41-62.
16. Friedman, H. J. Some Problems of Inpatient Management with Borderline Patients. *American Journal of Psychiatry,* 1969, 126:47-52.
17. Gunderson, J. G. and Singer, M. T. Defining Borderline Patients: An Overview. *American Journal of Psychiatry,* 1975, 132:1-10.
18. Friedman, H. J. Psychotherapy of Borderline Patients: The Influence of Theory on Technique. *American Journal of Psychiatry,* 1975, 132:1048-1052.
19. Carsar, D., 1979.
20. Pildis, M. J., Salzman, C., Soverow, G., and Wolf, J. G. Day Hospital Treatment of Borderline Patients: A Clinical Perspective. *American Journal of Psychiatry,* 1978, 135: 594-596.
21. Burnham, D. L., 1966.
22. Carsar, D., 1979.
23. Burnham, D. L., 1966.
24. Carsar, D., 1979.
25. Adler, G., 1973.
26. Hartocollis, P. (Ed.) *Borderline Personality Disorders,* New York: International Universities Press, Inc., 307-327, 1977.
27. Burnham, D. L., 1966.
28. Main, T. F., 1957.
29. Friedman, H. J., 1969.

30. Adler, G., 1973.

31. Hartocollis, P., 1977.

32. Gunderson, J., Kerr, J., and Woods, D. The Families of Borderlines—A Comparative Study. *Archives of General Psychiatry,* 1980, 37:27-33.

33. Wishnie, H. A., 1975.

34. Wishnie, H. A., 1975.

35. Friedman, H. J., 1969.

36. Lynch, V. J., and Lynch, M. T. Borderline Personality. *Perspectives in Psychiatric Care,* 1977, 15(2):72-75.

37. Masterson, J. Intensive Psychotherapy of the Adolescent with a Borderline Syndrome. In Silvano Arieti (Ed.), *American Handbook of Psychiatry,* New York: Basic Books, 1974, 250-263.

Early Treatment Planning for Hospitalized Severe Borderline Patients

Jerry M. Lewis, MD

This article explores several approaches to treatment planning for hospitalized patients with severe borderline pathology during the early or resistant phase of treatment. It recommends an open or team formulation of the patient's psychopathology, particularly utilizing staff countertransference feelings as one method of developing an initial hypothesis about the patient's self-system. In addition, the possible harmful effects of aggressive confrontation and interpretation are stressed and suggestions made to minimize the possibility that such interventions are experienced by the patients as staff assaults.

This article focuses on but a single, limited segment of treatment planning for hospitalized patients with severe borderline pathology: several activities found useful during the initial, or resistance, phase of hospitalization.

As used in this paper, severe borderline pathology is considered in a restricted sense, i.e., as a certain part of a continuum of personality organization rather than as a structure underlying a broad range of personality disorders. It is bounded at one end by psychotic character structures and, at the other, by narcissistic personality structures. Along the borderline continuum are several levels of personality organization of varying degrees of primitiveness. To maintain the focus of this presentation, however, many issues surround-

Dr. Lewis is psychiatrist-in-chief of Timberlawn Psychiatric Hospital in Dallas. His paper was originally presented at the Central Neuropsychiatric Hospital Association meeting in March 1982 in Chicago.

This article was originally published in *The Psychiatric Hospital, Journal of the National Association of Private Psychiatric Hospitals,* Vol. 13:4, Fall 1982, and is reprinted here with permission of the publisher.

ing the etiology, diagnosis, and treatment of patients with borderline personality disorders are not discussed.

Treatment planning refers to those processes used to translate clinical data into a system of interventions. The data are derived from multiple sources: the patient's history and physical examination, special tests and investigations, family assessment, exploratory and structured interviews, evaluation of the patient's behavior within the hospital, and staff affective responses to the patient. These diverse data are synthesized into an initial hypothesis, a clinical formulation emphasizing those biological, psychological, and social variables that, in concert, may explain the patient's behavior. The clinical formulation is a tentative set of assumptions that change as new data emerge.

The treatment planning process helps the clinician and the treatment team to move from cognitive understanding to action. It attempts to answer certain questions, for example, "If the patient's assaultive behavior is understood as reflecting these variables, what specific interventions will assist him both to modify and to control the behavior and encourage the early development of a treatment alliance?" The interventions should, therefore, derive directly from the clinical formulation, yet be sufficiently concrete and specific to be operationally useful to the nursing and activities personnel who spend hours each day with the patient and are often the initial recipients of his or her primitive projections. Although, inevitably, there is a trial-and-error component to this level of treatment planning, it is a far cry from general, diffuse statements ("form a treatment alliance") that have little operational usefulness and often reflect a response to mandated hospital record-keeping.

The observations on which this article is based have grown out of my experience as an intramural consultant to the treatment units of one psychiatric hospital. This experience has included interviewing both newly admitted patients and those who seem to be "stuck," or who present difficulties associated with staff conflict regarding appropriate intervention measures. In addition, as a consultant, I attend unit meetings, team meetings, and patient staffing conferences.

In order to define clearly the context in which the treatment planning activities have been found useful, it seems appropriate to sketch briefly the nature of the hospital treatment units and the types of patients treated. The units are comprised of from 16 to 44 patients. The larger units are served by several treatment teams, each of which includes an administrative psychiatrist, sufficient nursing personnel to provide intensive staff-patient interaction, usually a resident psychiatrist, a psychiatric social worker (who may assist several treatment teams), a clinical psychologist who also provides services to several teams, and an activities therapist. Individual psychotherapy is provided by staff members who usually are not members of the unit treatment team. Group and family therapy also are offered by staff members who may or may not be members of the unit treatment team. The ultimate responsibility for the patient's treatment program is firmly in the hands of the administrative psychiatrist, whose style of leadership varies with personality, experience, and theoretical orientation, although all share a commitment to psychoanalytic concepts. Of particular importance, however, are the unit treatment milieu and the development of a protreatment group process.[1] The unit milieu is considered an active therapeutic environment wherein much of the basic work of treatment occurs, not merely an essentially passive holding environment awaiting intrapsychic changes that occur only in individual psychotherapy. Basic personality change is fostered by a combination of all modalities—milieu and individual, group, and family therapies.

With rare exception, the patients have severe psychopathology and represent failures from outpatient treatment and one or more brief, crisis-oriented hospitalizations. Diagnostically, most are either chronically psychotic or manifest severe character pathology. The latter group includes patients with either borderline personality disorders or severe narcissistic personality disorders.

PHASES OF HOSPITAL TREATMENT

Masterson,[2] Rinsley,[3] and Brown[4] have described the hospital treatment of severe borderline disorders as occurring in three stages. This approach has a number of advantages as long as the treating clinician understands that a given patient's progression through the stages is never as clear and decisive as the authors' descriptions suggest, and that periodic regression, usually precipitated by transferential events, is the rule rather than the exception.

The initial stage is termed "testing" by Masterson, "resistance" by Rinsley, and "confusion and containment" by Brown. During this time a repetitive pattern of defensive behavior occurs which serves to protect the patient from the emergence of abandonment depression. Fears of engulfment and rage are also seen. Although individual differences are obvious, for many patients the stage is characterized more by anger presenting as sarcasm; argumentativeness; threats; manipulations; and, at the extreme, rage and persecutory anxiety. From a psychodynamic point of view, the patient is understood to be relying on a variety of projective mechanisms wherein internalized primitive "bad" object representations are projected to others. Much of the patient's behavior is seen as an attempt to control the projected "badness." Such projective mechanisms and other primitive defenses may lead to a common staff reaction: Unit staff members may internalize the projections and, in company with the understandable, realistic frustrations of dealing with the patient's behavior, feel that they are "bad" or, at the minimum, impotent. When this sequence is coupled with a rapid switch by the patient to an ego state characterized by sadness, loneliness, and emptiness, there is considerable staff confusion. Not only the patient, but staff members as well, may come to feel a lack of clarity of boundaries.

The second stage ("working through"[2], "introject work"[3], or "hopelessness and replacement"[4] is characterized by the patient's gradually giving up fantasies or reunion with a perfect object, the diminution of rage and projection, and the development of a more or less stable period of sadness with a pronounced quality of hopelessness. During this stage, unit staff may come to feel that the patient is "stuck" and is never going to get well. However, as the patient continues to work in psychotherapy and on the unit, internal objects are integrated, and higher order defenses replace more primitive ones. The final stage ("separation"[2], "resolution" [3], or "gratitude and concern" [4], involves the patient's separation from important objects in the hospital.

The growing body of data regarding borderline pathology and the effect of patient projections on hospital staff and structure must be complemented by increasing awareness of the effect of the staff and hospital structure on the patient's behavior. Three interrelated variables need emphasis: the characteristics of individual staff members, the organizational structure of the treatment team, and the nature of the patient group process.

Little is known beyond the level of impressions about personality characteristics of staff members who are able to work effectively with severe borderline patients. The exposure each day to hours of primitive projections results in considerable stress, perhaps making the role of the individual psychotherapist, with his or her time-limited contacts, seem enviable. Even among staff members who demonstrate mature levels of personality organization and a capacity for both empathic closeness and cognitive detachment, there is variation in the ability to work with severe borderline patients. One must accept primitive and often aggressive projections and manage them through understanding, without responding with actions that either retaliate or involve massive retreat from the patient. To accomplish this task requires, among other things, a strong sense of connectedness to an effectively functioning treatment team.

TREATMENT TEAM STRUCTURE

The organizational structure of the treatment team is a decisive factor in the establishment of a therapeutic milieu. The organizational structure comprises the repetitive interactional patterns that reflect the distribution of power and closeness within the team. Each treatment team has a basic organizational structure, which undergoes change, however, in response to changes in the larger hospital structure, changes in individual staff members, and changes in the patient group. Johansen has described these structural changes in treatment teams in response to a high level of neediness, rage, or other primitive affects from a critical mass of severe borderline patients.*

We are impressed with the usefulness of conceptualizing treatment team structure along a continuum originally reported in our study of family systems,[5] and described in some detail by Carson.** At the most functional end of this continuum are organizational structures characterized by firm but shared leadership, significant reliance on negotiation, clear individual boundaries, high levels of closeness, and flexible responses to stress. The next level of organizational structure is characterized by rigidity, reliance on a central dominating staff member, prohibitions against open expression of affect, intrastaff relationships involving either great distance or

---

*Johansen KH: The impact of patients with chronic character pathology upon the psychiatric hospital. Presented at the Central Neuropsychiatric Hospital Association Meeting, Chicago, March 1982.

**Carson DI: A hospital family-staff support system. Presented at the River Oaks Foundation Symposium, New Orleans, Louisiana, March 1978.

underlying conflict, and an emphasis on control. At the most dysfunctional end of the continuum are organizational structures that are either severely disorganized or undifferentiated in the sense that individual boundaries are blurred. Although many factors are involved in establishing the treatment team's basic structure, the relationship between the administrative psychiatrist-team leader and the head nurse is most often crucial. Their ability to evolve jointly a respectful, collaborative relationship in which differences of opinion are discussed openly often sets the tone of the entire team.

Hospital treatment teams may move back and forth between flexibility and rigidity or conflict; but, for the most part, periods of disorganization are brief and occur in response to severe stress. An undifferentiated treatment team structure, with its blurred boundaries, often isolates itself from the total hospital system, requiring intervention from outside the treatment team itself to recover complete function.

The third important contextual variable in understanding patient behavior is the patient group process. This process varies from periods of an active, shared, protreatment attitude in which the group is involved in daily supportive and confronting activities to periods of intense group resistance to any treatment activities. These periods are characterized by group silence, acting-out, shared manipulations, and a host of other antitreatment processes. An earlier publication details our efforts to augment the likelihood of prolonged periods of protreatment group processes.[1]

These brief descriptions are meant only to illustrate those forces that may invite certain behaviors, particularly in patients with unclear boundaries. For a patient with borderline pathology to be admitted to a treatment unit during a period of intense group resistance characterized by high levels of destructive behavior is quite provocative. When, in addition, there is associated treatment team rigidity and emphasis on automatic rules and controls, the situation grows even more complex. Such circumstances are very different from periods in which the patient group is working well together and the treatment team is firm but flexible in its response to changing circumstances.

Gunderson has emphasized the relationship of the borderline patient's manifest psychopathology and the current status of his or her relationship to a primary object.* However, he also suggests that

---

*Gunderson JG: Psychodynamic validation of borderline diagnosis. Presented at the 133rd Annual Meeting of the American Psychiatric Association, San Francisco, May 1980.

such a patient's fluctuating phenomenology can be related to the degree of external structure, which, at times, may have the same ameliorating effect as an object relationship. My observations of the borderline patients' manifest psychopathology (or shifting ego states) and treatment team structure confirm Gunderson's observations. Before such patients have established alliances with unit staff or individual psychotherapists, fluctuations in their manifest psychopathology often appear to be clearly correlated with treatment team structure. When this structure is basically flexible, warm, and supportive, many such patients experience themselves as sad, depressed, and lonely. They are conscious of wishes for intense connections to others. When the structure is experienced as over-controlling, frustrating, or conflicted, or there is an impending important loss (e.g., resignation of a staff member, discharge of a roommate) borderline patients without available primary objects feel vulnerable or angry and experience the unit as primitive, dangerous, and full of rage. When the unit structure is disorganized, however, some patients may panic or experience dissociative episodes or brief psychotic periods.

Gunderson suggests that borderline patients are responding to the availability of a primary object or the nature of the external structure. Often the sequence of events on a unit suggests such changes. At other times, however, the alteration in ego states seems to appear first within the patient, as if there were some type of central switching process, and the unit responds to the change in the patient. An angry, devaluing, difficult patient may drive staff and other patients away. If the patient suddenly appears sad, lonely, and reaches out to others, staff and patients alike may become warmer and more supportive. Although the correlation of patient ego state and structure of the treatment team seems clear, I cannot always be certain about which comes first. Perhaps it is best to recall Forrester's injunction that in complex systems the occurrence of two events close in time does not necessarily suggest causality, but, rather, may mean that both were caused by another yet undiscovered event.[9]

TREATMENT PLANNING

Many aspects of treatment planning will not be discussed in this paper. Rather, the focus is restricted to a few clinical activities that have seemed particularly useful for this group of patients during the early stage of hospitalization. The problems that must be addressed include a realistic need to contain such patients and prevent injury either to themselves or to others. A second problem is the need to establish an early treatment alliance between the patient and unit staff. A third is the need to deal with an array of staff feelings about the patient, frequently including shared staff confusion.

That treatment planning for a hospitalized borderline patient begins with construction of a clinical formulation is, of course, apparent. The advantage of encouraging the entire treatment team to participate in constructing the formulation must be emphasized. Most often the psychiatrist (administrative psychiatrist or individual therapist) takes the lead, although other members of the treatment team may do so occasionally. This leader needs to encourage the participation of all members of the treatment team but at the same time have a broader and deeper knowledge of the subject material and act as teacher. Such clinical leadership—based on the ability to listen and to synthesize the observations of others—is not, of course, possessed by all psychiatrists, nor is it necessarily lacking in professionals from other mental health disciplines. Indeed, a professional with these leadership qualities does not compete with other members of the team but acknowledges, welcomes, and uses their special expertise. Although it may be that in other settings other structures work well, in the setting described a psychiatrist takes the responsibility of leadership.

The advantages of constructing the clinical formulation in a team setting rather than privately in the mind of either the administrative psychiatrist or therapist seem clear: Doing so provides the psychiatrist with a wider range of observations, and richer clinical data are available with which to construct the formulation.

A second advantage is that, to the extent that team members participate in construction of the formulation, they will consider it their own, using it as a base from which to intervene in the patient's behavior. It is impossible *not* to have a set of assumptions about the patient's behavior, and constructing the clinical formulation as a team increases the likelihood of a shared model and a more consistent approach to interventions. In this way, the "open" process of constructing a formulation minimizes the likelihood that the milieu is perceived by the patient as conflicted or disorganized.

Another advantage is the increased learning from each other that goes on in this type of team meeting. Although the psychiatrist may carry the major teaching load, he or she also learns from the special knowledge and skills of colleagues. When this reciprocal process moves well, it augments the growth of mutuality and cohesion on the treatment team and does so while maintaining an appropriate focus—understanding and responding to patients' needs.

It is important to emphasize that construction of a clinical formulation is essentially an inductive process. To provide leadership in this task requires a capacity for synthesizing data of markedly different levels of complexity. Information from the patient's history, data regarding the current functioning of the patient's family, and observations about the patient's initial response to the treatment team and other patients on the unit are but examples of sources of data used in constructing a clinical formulation.

Two additional sources of data which are valuable in treatment planning for patients with severe borderline disorders are obtaining staff members' affective responses to the patient and conducting a particular type of exploratory interview. Staff affective responses are a source of information which is important in constructing a clinical formulation, and sharing these responses should be routine. The cathartic advantage in such sharing should never outweigh its purpose, that the treatment team use these shared feelings in the service of understanding the patient better.

SOURCES OF COUNTERPRODUCTIVE AFFECT

Although there are numerous sources of counter-productive staff affect directed at patients, three seem of particular importance. One grows more or less naturally out of the daily tribulations of managing and trying to help these frequently difficult patients. A second source reflects intrateam tensions and conflicts, which lead to feelings that are projected onto the patient group or onto a particular patient, making the recipient a scapegoat.

When these two sources of staff affect are detected and understood, the treatment team is freed to deal with the third source of staff affect: important countertransference responses to the patient. Here the focus is on those aspects of countertransference which concern internalization by staff of patients' projections rather than the projection by staff of the remnants of their own earlier object relationships. At times, clarification of these projections can provide the treatment team with a cognitive map of the patient's internal objective representations, which can be helpful in constructing a clinical formulation.

Frequently one of two clinical situations is noted. In one, all members of the treatment team develop much the same counter-transference response to a patient. Each staff member experiences a similar kind of anger, warmth, or other feelings. In short, there is no evidence of splitting. However, changes in the patient's ego state, with consequent change in the content of the patient's projections, may lead to a clear shift in the nature of the shared staff countertransference response. Understanding these changes can be of great help in planning interventions. The second type of presentation involves splitting. In this instance, members of the treatment team divide into two camps that correspond to the patient's projection of unintegrated polarities. As a consequence, one group, for example, sees the patient as helpless and needy, whereas the other group sees the patient as hostile and dangerous.

One function of the clinical formulation involves locating the patient on the continuum of personality organization, i.e., identifying how primitive or, conversely, better integrated is the personality structure. Although there is considerable debate about whether such determinations can be made other than through an evolving transference to an individual psychotherapist, I have found that an interview exploring how the patient experiences himself or herself may offer valuable insights regarding the cohesiveness of the patient's self-system. The patient's use of splitting usually becomes clear in such an interview, and clues regarding cohesiveness of the self can often be inferred from exploring whether the patient experiences two or more distinctly different ego states. These very different ways of experiencing the self and the world rarely occur concurrently; rather, they are experienced consecutively. Commonly there are but two ego states: One is essentially depressive, and the other is paranoid:

> A 14-year old girl having many features of a severe borderline disorder was still in the resistance stage of treatment after several months. Her behavior was alternately needy and raging. She was interviewed during a room restriction, occasioned by the failure of other interventions to alter her angry, aggressive, and manipulative behavior.
>
> In response to the explorations of how she felt inside, she described herself as sad and intensely lonely. The loneliness was associated with a conscious longing for (and image of) her mother. Later in the interview she described a very different experience of herself that, for a few hours, punctuated the days

of sadness and intense loneliness. During this second ego state she was free of those affects and, most important, if restricted to her room, felt safe. Exploration of this feeling led to the disclosure of a clear projective system in which she felt that she was under dangerous attack from the nursing staff. Those nurses who, at other times, were perceived as most nurturing were, during these intervals, seen as most threatening. If room restriction did not isolate her from those "dangerous nurses," she could not identify factors that led to these dramatic changes.

The demonstration (or report) of such shifting ego states suggests a tenuous self-system. Some patients, however, are resistant to this type of exploration, particularly during the early weeks of hospitalization; therefore, the inability to demonstrate such shifting ego states does not prove a cohesive self-system.

It is valuable to conduct such interviews in the presence of members of the treatment team. Their understanding of borderline pathology becomes clearer, and their capacity to relate the results of the exploration to intervention efforts is often augmented.

I would like to emphasize the usefulness in treatment planning of a clear delineation of the borderline patient's projective mechanisms. In particular, familiarity with Ogden's clarification of the process of projective identification, precisely because it bridges the gap between intrapsychic and interpersonal phenomena, can be crucial for both staff understanding and the planning of specific interventions.[7,8]

CONFRONTATION AND INTERPRETATION

In addition to the advantages of an "open" clinical formulation, I would like to address the role of staff confrontation and interpretation in planning treatment. My thesis is that treatment planning should emphasize the sparing use of confrontation and interpretation by the treatment team during the early resistance stage of a patient's hospital treatment. Although there is much general agreement about the necessity and usefulness of these interventions, our follow-up study of formerly hospitalized adolescents suggests that these techniques, particularly when used aggressively and before a treatment alliance has been established, are recalled years later by former patients as hostile assaults.[9] Former patients, independent of treatment outcome and overall feelings about their hospital treatment, vividly recall the painful feelings consequent to confrontations and interpretations, especially during the early weeks of hospitalization. Soll, in a related discussion of individual psychotherapy and psychoanalysis with such patients, stresses the need for much preliminary work in order to minimize the possible narcissistic injury brought about by interpretations.* Therefore, the mandate to treatment planners is to find gentler intervention techniques for this stage, ways of facilitating exploration and guiding the therapeutic work which avoid the possible damage of confrontation and interpretation.

First, however, it is necessary to distinguish between patients' verbal and motor behavior during this stage of treatment. It is, of course, axiomatic that the staff must protect the patient and others from harmful, aggressive motor behavior. The unit rules and consequences for physical assault must be absolutely clear. Treatment teams, however, must develop a tolerance for verbal expressions of hostility. Although certain categories of verbal behavior (e.g., direct threats) may be explicitly forbidden, the unit must serve to some degree as a holding environment for the projections of such patients. The issue of how much and what kind of verbal behavior to allow is complex, and it is important that each treatment team address its own holding capacity and attempt to reach a consensus. There is no absolute level of tolerance which works for all treatment teams or for a particular treatment team at all times.

An important aspect of the use of confrontation and interpretation is that such interventions appear to have reduced destructive potential when they come from peers rather than staff. Most patients are somewhat accepting of verbal feedback from fellow patients, particularly if it comes from several of them. During periods of patients' protreatment group process there is an effective balance between peer confrontation-interpretation and empathic support. Efforts of the treatment team to assist patients in achieving a protreatment group process are enhanced, therefore, in that the patient group assumes a significant part of the work of confrontation and interpretation.

---

*Soll M: Techniques of interpretation in neurotic versus more primitive personality structure, parts I & II. Presented at the Timberlawn Psychiatric Hospital Lecture Series, Dallas, February 2 and 9, 1982.

Another principle concerns the technique of confrontation and interpretation. Every effort must be made to develop a style of *respectful* intervention. Understanding the internal superior-inferior and aggressor-victim polarities of such patients often helps unit staff. To know that within the overtly demeaning, devaluating, and omnipotent patient resides a vulnerable, inferior portion of his or her self-system may help the staff develop some degree of tolerance.

A confrontation or interpretation has a greater chance of helping (and less chance of harming) if it has certain structural features. Interventions directed against specific incidents or sets of behavior (i.e., circumscribed) and delivered in a matter-of-fact way are less likely to hurt than are those addressed to a broad segment of the patient's behavior or character as a whole (i.e., diffuse) and given in a hostile or harsh way. Of course, intrusive statements ("you enjoy making me mad") are to be avoided.

We have been experimenting with the use of techniques designed to reduce the treatment team's reliance on confrontation and interpretation during this early stage of resistance. A promising, but certainly not original, technique has been to involve the patient in monitoring some aspect of his or her behavior. Although many patients with severe borderline pathology describe various ego states, most are much less aware of the relationship patterns that flow from these ego states. These relationship patterns often produce behavior in others which sustains the ego state. A borderline patient in a paranoid rage, for example, may provoke others to fear an attack. As a consequence, staff may become overly cautious and retreat, thereby increasing the patient's sense that "something is up—they are treating me as if I am different." This situation may lead to increased rage and, ultimately, result in a staff decision to control the patient physically, which, in turn, adds fuel to the paranoid fire.

Several approaches to such a patient are feasible. One is to help the patient set up a daily chart on which to record briefly the main feeling tone for that day or nursing shift. Patients use such terms as "sad," "lonely," "angry," and "feeling good." In another column of the chart the patient is asked to write several sentences describing the most intense, interpersonal experience that occurred during the same time period. This type of chart, kept by the patient and reviewed each day by a member of the treatment team, allows the patient to begin to establish some rough correlations between internal states and interpersonal relationships.

A second approach is to define, in collaboration with the patient, several levels of anger and have the patient chart daily these anger levels and his or her perceptions of the response from staff and others. This type of prescribed activity appears to help, first because it is a joint staff-patient activity that strongly underscores the collaborative nature of treatment, and, second, because it augments the development of an observing ego, particularly in relating the nature or intensity of internal states to changes in the surrounding interpersonal context. As such, these interventions may help the patient to understand his or her projective mechanisms. In addition, these activities appear to reduce the need for confrontation and interpretation; and, although these interventions continue to be important, staff members appear less likely to engage in escalating power conflicts with patients.

CONCLUSION

The treatment of severe borderline patients is a major focus of many psychotherapeutically oriented hospitals. Follow-up study suggests that many such patients make dramatic and lasting changes if treatment is intensive and continues over a sufficient period of time. However, we need to continue searching for ways to make hospital treatment even more effective and, if possible, of shorter duration. Part of this complex problem is the need of the unit staff to share a clinical formulation that makes both the patient's behavior and staff affective responses understandable and that offers the staff a number of intervention options that carry less risk of being experienced as assaultive by the patient during the crucial early period of hospitalization. This article describes several clinical processes that address these concerns—an "open" clinical formulation and involvement of the patient in self-monitoring.

REFERENCES

1. Lewis JM, Gossett JT, King J, Carson DI: Development of a protreatment group process among hospitalized adolescents, in Adolescent Psychiatry, Vol 2. Edited by Feinstein SC, Giovacchini PL. New York, Basic Books, 1975

2. Masterson, J: Treatment of the Borderline Adolescent: A Developmental Approach. New York, John Wiley and Sons, Inc, 1972

3. Rinsley DB: Theory and practice of intensive residential treatment of patients with borderline personality disorders. Psychiatr Q 42:611-618, 1968

4. Brown LJ: The therapeutic milieu in the treatment of patients with borderline personality disorders. Bull Menninger Clinic 45(5):377-394, 1981

5. Lewis JM, Beavers WR, Gossett JT, Phillips VA: No Single Thread: Psychological Health in Family Systems. New York, Brunner/Mazel, 1977

6. Forrester JW: Urban Dynamics, Boston, MIT Press, 1969

7. Ogden TH: Projective identification in psychiatric hospital treatment. Bull Menninger Clinic 45(4):317-333, 1981

8. Ogden TH: On projective identification. Int J Psychoanal 60(3):357-373, 1979

9. Gossett JT, Lewis JM, Barnhart FD, Phillips VA: The adolescent treatment assessment project: lessons learned in process. NAPPH J 8(3):26-30, 1976

Update of Borderline Disorders in Children

Paulina F. Kernberg, MD

Borderline personality disorder in children can be considered to be a definable entity and diagnostic category significantly associated with minimal brain dysfunction and depression. Borderline personality organization cuts across the diagnostic categories of neuroses, psychoses, and organic disorders. Descriptive symptoms are in themselves not telling; the most reliable criteria for making the diagnosis of borderline personality are the children's sudden shifts in levels of functioning, lack of a sense of identity, inability to accept responsibility for their own actions, and inability to experience pleasure in play. The characteristics of treatment and especially of psychoanalytic psychotherapy of these patients are outlined.

Until relatively recent years, the term borderline was not generally applied to children. There was hesitation about attributing a personality disorder to children between six and 12 years old; children of that age were either neurotic, psychotic, or suffered from an organic disorder of some sort. The current trend is to draw a distinction between childhood psychosis and borderline conditions. A delineation of the latter has been made by Pine, Chethik, and Rinsley, among others.[1,2,3]

The Diagnostic and Statistical Manual of Mental Disorders Third Edition (DSM-III)[4] does not contain a category for borderline personality disorder in children; nor does it contain a category for any other personality disorder in children, thereby perpetuating the old-fashioned assumption that children do not suffer from personality disorders.

Dr. Kernberg is director of child and adolescent psychiatry, The New York Hospital-Westchester Division, Cornell University Medical Center; associate professor of psychiatry, Cornell University Medical College; a training and supervising adult and child analyst, Columbia University Center for Psychoanalytic Training and Research; and a member of the Editorial Board of *The Psychiatric Hospital.*

This article was originally published in *The Psychiatric Hospital, Journal of the National Association of Private Psychiatric Hospitals* Vol. 13:4, Fall 1982, and is reprinted here with permission of the publisher.

THE CLINICAL PICTURE

Clinical evidence shows, however, that the syndrome does exist. We have, for the past ten years, been treating children whose clinical picture is distinctly different from the pictures presented by neuroses, psychoses, or organic syndromes. These children present clinical manifestations that correspond to what Kernberg,[5] has described as the borderline personality organization in adults and adolescents. In agreement with Kernberg, I conceive of the borderline condition as cutting across the usual diagnostic categories of neuroses, psychoses, and organic states and as differing from these categories both quantitatively and qualitatively.

These children might suffer from obsessions, phobias, compulsions, or hysterical states; but these symptoms are in themselves not telling. Nor are the symptoms of poor impulse control, inability to control behavior, especially aggressive behavior, or a low tolerance for frustration and depression, any/or all of which may be present.

The most reliable criteria for making the diagnosis of borderline personality organization are the children's sudden shifts in levels of functioning, their inability to accept responsibility for their own actions, and lack of a sense of identity: They do not feel themselves as firmly belonging to one gender or the other, nor are they sure of what they can or cannot do.

By the time the normal child is six years old, he can be expected to be able to differentiate himself from other people realistically and to display a beginning sense of autonomy. Although he still shows some ambivalence around dependency issues, he can tolerate being separated from his mother without becoming anxious. He also knows the difference between right and wrong without her having to tell him. He has the rudiments, or more, of reality testing; is aware of the differential qualities of other people; and, to some extent, of their needs. He can express such feelings as shame, guilt, joy, and love. Above all, the normal or neurotic child of six years can recognize his own attributes and roles—he has a sense of who and what he is, both socially and sexually.

Our normal six-year-old might, for example, say, "I am a boy; I am good at baseball; I like guns. I live with my family near my school. Tomorrow I am going to play baseball with Johnny and Dick. Sometimes my parents punish me, but not too often."

A borderline child of the same age or older, however, will say (indeed, has said), "I am Superman. I can fly . . . I can't fly. If I did jump like Superman, I might get hurt and a policeman would have to help me.'' The borderline child cannot say what his attributes are and rarely conveys a sense of "me-ness." He cannot predict future behavior on the basis of past performance.

Yet, these borderline children do not suffer from delusions, do not behave in bizarre fashion, and display no disorganization of thought. Their thinking may not always be logical; but, if challenged to clarify their statements, they are, unlike the psychotic child, able to do so. And if they do lose contact with reality, the loss is transitory, lasting sometimes only minutes, other times a few hours, or, at most, a few days.

The children I am describing do hallucinate—their hallucinations are usually auditory or visual, consisting of voices or apparitions commanding them to behave badly or to harm themselves. The hallucinations are typically transitory, are not accompanied by intense anxiety, and are usually triggered by some untoward external event. It is well to remember that neurotic children also hallucinate, and that, given the circumstances, children generally hallucinate more easily than do adults.[6]

Another typical characteristic of the borderline child is his inability to experience pleasure in play. Play is compulsive, at best without development and resolution of fantasy themes. Interruption of play under the impact of anxiety is frequent. These children prefer structured games, either table games or ball games, where control of fantasy is kept in abeyance.

The nature of their interpersonal relationships further distinguishes the children under survey here. The borderline children want to be in control. Because they are demanding and manipulative, their peers do not want to have anything to do with them. And so they are caught in a terrible bind because, while they cannot get along with others, they cannot tolerate being alone. Even minor stress disorganizes them; but, unlike psychotic children, if they lapse into a psychotic state, the duration is brief.

When we speak of borderline personality organization, we are speaking about a defect in ego development. If ego development depends on perception, attention, and memory, and if these functions are defective due to organicity, then the mental representations—the concepts of the self and others—will be distorted. Thus the child with minimal brain dysfunction will certainly find it harder to negotiate the developmental tasks required in order to have a realistic idea of himself and of significant others. The difficulties will be enhanced by the absence of positive feedback. Because the child cannot respond appropriately to the mother's cues, both mother and child live in a state of constant frustration. Frustration produces hostile aggression. Hostile aggression leads to negative feedback from the environment. And so on.

I realize that in using the term minimal brain dysfunction I am again disagreeing with *DSM-III,* which employs the diagnosis of attention deficit disorder. I find this term too limiting: Minimal brain dysfunction accounts for a variety of organic deficits in addition to attention deficit, all of which may impinge on the child's early development. Furthermore, *DSM-III* places attention deficit disorder in Axis I, and I believe it belongs in Axis II, insofar as attention deficit disorders are frequently associated with learning disabilities and the early development of the child is bound to be affected by the presence of attention deficit and learning disorders.

The borderline child with minimal brain dysfunction is particularly prone to being depressed. These children have, according to Wender,[8] a primary deficit in experiencing affect and a lowered sensitivity to reinforcement so that they fail to heed cautions, requests, and demands. Further, because of their relative difficulty in experiencing pleasure, they require more sensation, are harder to satiate, and are bored more easily than normal children. At the same time, they require more than ordinary disciplinary action owing to their impulsiveness. Hence, they fail to meet parental expectations, which diminishes their self-esteem, which in turn increases their depressiveness. Add to all these considerations the burden of not enjoying the satisfaction afforded by the sense of mastery, or from establishing gratifying relationships with others, and the chronic depressiveness of these children becomes very understandable.

TREATMENT CONSIDERATIONS

Treatment objectives are to establish in the child a firm sense of identity and an equally firm sense of the child's object world. We aim to improve his capacity to relate to others in a realistic manner and to function more autonomously. Our approach is multimodal: *a)* We provide a stable and predictable environment, either through hospitalization or through active work at the family level. (Most of the families need help to organize their routines and interactions.) *b)* We prescribe, especially when the child is hyperactive and destructive, a trial of methylphenidate or dextroamphetamine for the minimal brain dysfunction component. The rationale behind administering drugs is to improve the child's capacity to benefit from psychological treatment. To the same end, imipramine may be used for relieving depression. *c)* We offer remedial therapy for any learning disability stemming from organic factors. Attention to the deficit aspect has a reinforcing effect in that an improvement in school performance will encourage the child to feel better about himself. Consequently, his relationships with peers improve because decreasing his anxiety also decreases his coercive and manipulative behavior. *d)* Finally, we treat the child with individual psychoanalytically oriented psychotherapy. (With the youngest children, problems stemming from separation may require conjoint therapy of the mother-child pair. More often than not, we find the child more ready to leave the mother than the mother is to leave the child.)

The child is seen twice or three times a week for a period that can be as long as three years. The therapist's role is crucial in that he or she is the instrument through which the child will develop an integrated sense of himself and of others. The child is then able to acquire new experiences in the external world of friends, family, and other interests. Settlage's description[9] of the mother's affirming functions cannot be improved on as a guide for the therapist in these cases: "[The child] needs her affirmation of him in changing and expanding his sense of self and identity, her validation of his continuing importance to her, of his developing skills and abilities, of his urges and feelings and their acceptability and manageability, and of the continuity of his old and new self in her eyes." In working with a mother-child dyad, the therapist systematically explores and brings out the anxiety evoked when a child begins to separate himself psychologically from his mother—the fears of being abandoned or destroyed. These fears need to be verbalized to both the mother and the child.

The kind of anxiety the borderline children experience is typical. It is intense and diffuse, reduces the child to a state of panic, and results in a noticeable drop in level of functioning. Even minor provocation can disorganize these children. They are subject to temper tantrums, will physically attack others, and frequently present suicidal ideation or acts. If they do lapse into a psychotic state, the state will typically have a paranoid flavor.

Our diagnostic armamentarium includes a full battery of tests: WISC; the Wechsler Intelligence; Binet; the Wide Range Achievement Test, tests for psycholinguistic abilities, auditory and visual discrimination; and other specific language tests are selectively administered to children entering our service. More systematic observations are obtained by the use of the Connor Teacher Rating Scale for evaluation of hyperactivity throughout time. We find out as much as possible about the parents—especially their childhood history. We are also careful to inquire about perinatal complications—all with the idea of exploring possible organic factors. Reports from teachers are important, especially in connection with finding out how the child functions academically and learning more about his interpersonal relations.

ETIOLOGICAL CONSIDERATIONS

Our current knowledge of the etiology of borderline conditions is still tentative. The most interesting and relevant set of hypotheses is Mahler's developmental theory,[7] particularly her description of the separation individuation process. According to Mahler, the process occurs during the first three years of life: The infant proceeds from an autistic phase through a symbiotic phase and a separation-individuation phase to a stage she calls "on the road to [emotional] object constancy." When development during the rapproachment subphase of separation-individuation is disordered or unsuccessful, borderline phenomena may result. This rapproachement subphase, usually completed by the end of the second year, includes the task of integrating the concepts of the self and of significant others. Abnormal mother-infant interaction during separation-individuation produces excessive and pathological conflicts in the child—conflicts between love and hate, between autonomy and dependence. The child's conflicts cause him to behave in ways that perpetuate the abnormal mother-infant interactions, and they spill over and contaminate the child's other interpersonal relations.

Thus, abnormal family interactions can interfere with the separation-individuation process and, thereby, contribute to establishing borderline personality organization. Another contributing factor might well be organic.

BORDERLINE PERSONALITY ORGANIZATION
AND MINIMAL BRAIN DYSFUNCTION

In the course of diagnostic testing of the children on our service, we noticed what seemed to us an extraordinarily high incidence of organicity. This finding, together with the high incidence of inattention, impulsiveness, and hyperactivity which were observed in children we were diagnosing as borderline, alerted us to the possibility that these children were also suffering from minimal brain dysfunction. We subsequently found that a significant percentage of both outpatient and inpatient children were suffering from both minimal brain dysfunction and borderline personality organization and that the two syndromes clearly overlapped. The precise nature of the relationship between the two syndromes is more ambiguous. I suspect that a minimal brain dysfunction would predispose a child to developing a borderline personality organization.

If the child suffers from minimal brain dysfunction, a constant clarification of how the child perceives the therapist and the therapist's interventions is essential. In this way, the child is acknowledging his difficulty around attention, memory, or sequencing—whatever the deficit may be. This carefully engineered clarification also enables the therapist to accommodate the level and speed of his speech to the child's specific needs. Moreover, as intuitively described by Frosch[10] and Greenson,[11] this type of intervention increases the understanding between the patient and therapist. Both can acknowledge that the child's distorted perceptions of the therapist may be due not only to resistance to treatment but also to difficulties in attention and memory, as well as in perceiving social interactions.

In addition, it is important when the picture includes minimal brain dysfunction to clarify the nature of the deficits and their possible impact on the child's adaptive capacities, as well as the possible ways of compensating for these deficits. By talking realistically about the child's deficits, the therapist enables the child to acknowledge the deficit, to share the knowledge with a trusted person, and to grieve. The child can then elaborate and resolve fantasy systems in connection with his deficits. These fantasies usually are concerned with guilt or the child's feeling that he has been bad. They have thus contributed to the child's low self-esteem. Now the child has a chance to gain mastery through compensatory mechanisms. A child whose visual memory was deficient, for example, can resort to writing words; a child with auditory deficits in memory can supplement them with visual input.

Clearly, the principal therapeutic technique employed in what I have been describing is that of clarification. Clarification implies that the material being dealt with is preconscious.[12] Clarification is as unlike confronting a patient with unconscious wishes or impulses as it is unlike "supporting" the patient by ignoring or minimizing the realities of his situation.

Clarification extends to the primitive defense mechanisms as the child employs these in the therapeutic situation: splitting, projection, devaluation, omnipotence, or denial. Similarly, the therapist clarifies the contradictory ego states as the child experiences them, explaining what lies behind them. If the child acts out, this too is given attention.

In advocating clarification as a therapeutic technique, I cannot stress too strongly the need for the therapist to exercise great care in how he times and phrases his interventions. It is essential that he feel along with the child; it is equally essential that he not act out if the child provokes him. The therapist remembers that despite the borderline patient's tendency to distort reality, he does have the capacity to test reality. A second general principle of treatment is to stress the here and now, that is, to give preference to interactions within the sessions as they unfold through the relationship with the therapist and through play activities rather than interventions having to do with the patient's past history. Interventions having to do with the past will be far less effective for a child who, especially in the first stages of treatment, has no integrated concept of himself or others and no sense of continuity about his life.

The adjustment to the family requires that the child have a realistic perception of himself and his contributions to his parents' behavior and also a realistic perception of the parents' personalities. It is not infrequent to see incidents of overt maternal rejection in these cases. This too must be clarified. If grief over family deficits is dealt with in therapy, the child may then be free to find and recognize the positive aspects still existing in his parents and also to seek out and accept other adults to supplement these missing parental functions.

The therapist deals with the child's difficulties in relation to peers by articulating how the child behaves in the therapeutic situation vis-à-vis the therapist. This procedure, I should add, contains risks, for the therapist might act out the anger these children can so easily provoke.

Any potential disruptive experience, impending hospitalization, for example, or impending parental divorce, needs to be anticipated and verbalized since these children lack signal anxiety and thus are prone to falling into panic states; these states of panic are enhanced by the omnipotent and magical thinking characteristic of these children.

CONCLUSION

In conclusion, I am suggesting that borderline personality disorder in children seems to be a definable entity and diagnostic category, significantly associated with minimal brain dysfunction and depression. Therapeutic intervention requires a careful assessment of organic and psychological determinants in order to institute an appropriate treatment plan.

I am further suggesting that the psychological segment of treatment be psychoanalytically oriented psychotherapy that focuses on clarification, with the aim of fortifying the child's sense of reality. Included is making the child aware of his deficits.

REFERENCES

1. Pine F: On the concept "borderline" in children: a clinical essay, in The Psychoanalytic Study of the Child 29. New Haven, Yale University Press, 1974

2. Chethik M: The borderline child, in *Basic Handbook of Child Psychiatry*. Edited by Noshpitz JD. New York, Basic Books, 1979

3. Rinsley DB: Diagnosis and treatment of borderline and narcissistic children and adolescents, in *Treatment of the Severly Disturbed Adolescent*. Edited by Rinsley DB. New York, Jason Aronson, 1980

4. American Psychiatric Association: Diagnostic and Statistical Manual of Mental Disorders, 3rd ed (DSM-III). Washington, DC, APA, 1980

5. Kernberg O: Borderline Conditions and Pathological Narcissism. New York, Jason Aronson, 1975

6. Coren HZ, Saldinger JS: Visual hallucinosis in children: a report of two cases in The Psychoanalytic Study of the Child 22. New York, International Universities Press, 1967

7. Mahler M, Pine F, Bergman A: The Psychological Birth of the Human Infant. New York, Basic Books, 1975

8. Wender P: Minimal Brain Dysfunction in Children. New York, Wiley & Sons, 1971

9. Settlage CF: The psychoanalytic understanding of narcissistic and borderline personality: advances in developmental theory. J Am Psychoanal Assoc 25:805-833, 1977

10. Frosch J: Techniques in regard to some specific ego deficits in the treatment of borderline patients. Psychiatr Q: 45:216-220, 1971

11. Greenson RR: The struggle against identification. J Am Psychoanal Assoc 2:200-217, 1954

12. Bibring GL: Psychoanalysis and the dynamic psychotherapies. J Am Psychoanal Assoc 2:745-770, 1954